My Mindful Moments

Name: _____

Year: _____   Age: _____

Contents

Me & My Year

Feelings & Emotions

Life Skills, Values & Personal Qualities

Unwind

Introduction

Life is full of opportunities, experiences and challenges that impact each and every one of us differently. As we journey through life, we can find ourselves in struggle. We can find others in struggle. Our understanding, environment and skillset are essential in managing these effectively. *My Mindful Moments* is a life skills toolkit filled with reflection activities to journal and deepen our understanding of ourselves and the world. It focuses on habitual awareness and growth mindset to promote balanced lives filled with competence, resilience and contentment.

This workbook is designed to create purposeful wellbeing for children and young people- a place to find strength, insight, connection and inspiration. It can be completed independently or collaboratively with an adult, to boost positive relationships with mental health. As we grow, our thoughts, feelings and experiences change too.

My Mindful Moments has the most impact when inputted daily, no matter how small the contribution. Completing a new *My Mindful Moments* workbook every year or two promotes relative, authentic reflection on your development- reminding yourself just how far you have come.

You are amazing. You matter. You can make a difference.

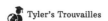

Wellbeing

Wellbeing is a multifaceted term: it has many vital components and influences. Generally, it describes the quality of our lives and our state of being happy, comfortable and healthy mentally, psychologically, socially, emotionally and spiritually. Everything we think, believe, feel and do affects our wellbeing. Positive wellbeing is improved through connecting, learning, being active, giving and mindfulness.

Mental Health

Mental health is a state of wellbeing that affects how we think, feel and act- this can be positive or negative. It determines how we connect with others, our decision-making, our self-regulation and how we deal with adversity. It exists on a continuum, encompassing our psychological, emotional and social wellbeing. Mental health is paramount throughout our entire lives- it can impact anything and everything.

Mindfulness

Mindfulness defines our ability to be fully present in the current moment- awareness of where we are, what we are doing, how we feel and what we are thinking. It is a quality we are all born with; the challenge is often being able to access it and allow it to be transformative. Mindfulness begins and ends in the body, purely and peacefully accepting ourselves and living in the moment.

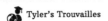 Tyler's Trouvailles

Why are they important?

 They reduce feelings of depression, stress, anxiety and loneliness.

 They affect how we learn and grow as individuals, deepening our understanding and knowledge of ourselves, others and the world.

 They enable us to overcome difficulties and achieve our goals.

 They allow us to recognise and respond appropriately to our feelings and emotions.

 They provide clarity, informing and supporting our choices.

 They affect our ability to connect and develop positive relationships with others.

 They promote acceptance, resilience, respect and gratitude.

Growth Mindset

Having a growth mindset defines our ability to change, learn and develop. When we have a growth mindset, we see challenges as opportunities to grow. We can achieve anything with belief, effort and the right strategies to support us.

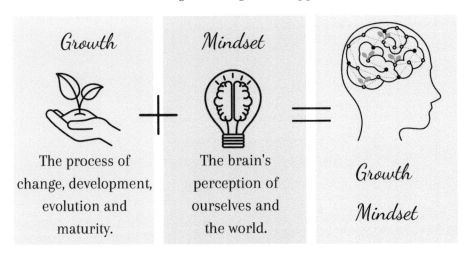

Growth

The process of change, development, evolution and maturity.

Mindset

The brain's perception of ourselves and the world.

Growth Mindset

Fixed Mindset

A fixed mindset is the opposite of a growth mindset. It defines the belief that our personal qualities and abilities are fixed. For example, believing change and development is impossible. This can sabotage our happiness, success and health.

Fixed Mindset

"I give up, it's too hard."

"I stick to what I know."

"I will never improve."

Growth Mindset

"Challenges help me grow."

"I like to try new things."

"I will keep trying my best."

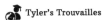

How can you support a growth mindset?
Write your ideas around the image.

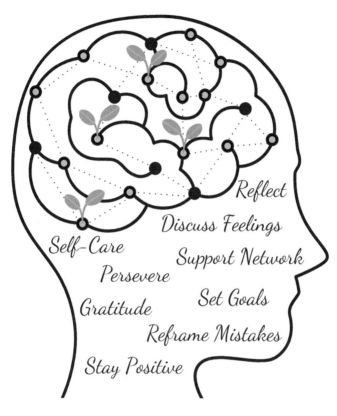

What do you think a growth mindset looks, sounds and feels like?

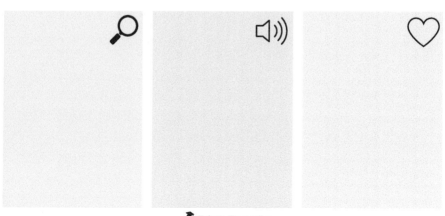

Me & My Year

This is Me

HELLO
my name is

Draw a self-portrait.

My Family

Draw and label everyone in your family.
Remember- not all families are the same, they are all unique and
wonderful in their own way.

My Special Day

My Birthday is on

_____

Draw or write your best memories of today.

Design your dream birthday cake.

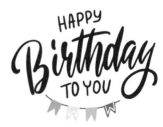

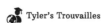

Birthdays

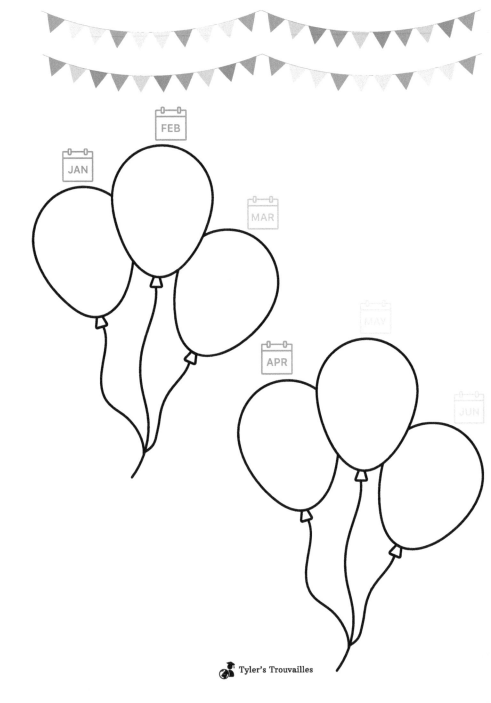

Birthdays give everyone a special day to celebrate their life, growth and achievements.

Write the names and birthdates of your family and friends in the balloons.
This will remind you to spread extra kindness on their special day.

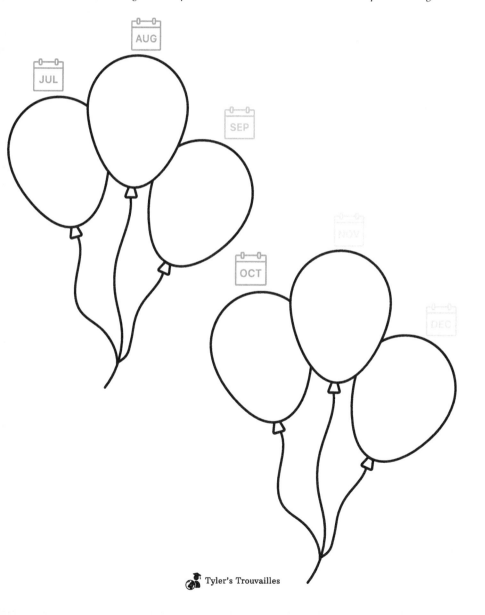

My Favourite Things

Use the alphabet to create a record of all of your favourite things- the things you like the most!

A

B

C

D

E

F

G

H

Things to consider:
- *Food*
- *Places*
- *People*
- *Books*
- *Subjects*
- *TV/Films*
- *Events*
- *Experiences*
- *Hobbies*
- *Sports*
- *Animals*
- *Music*
- *Seasons*
- *Colours*

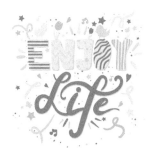

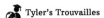 Tyler's Trouvailles

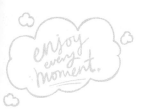

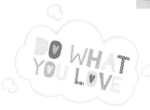

I
J
K
L
M
N
O
P

R
S
T
U
V
W
X
Y
Z

My Library

*Record the books you
have read this year by
writing their titles on
the book spines!*

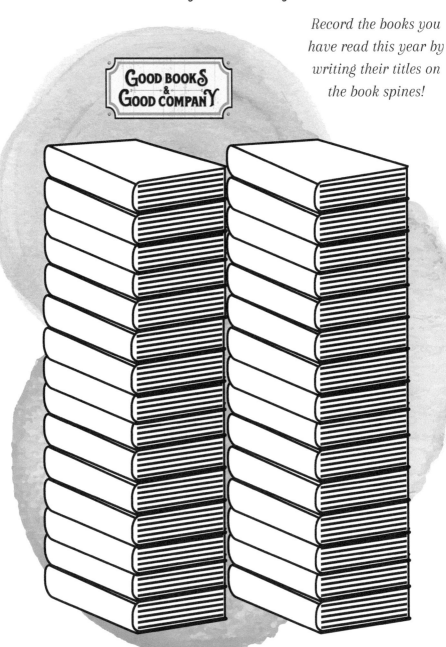

GOOD BOOKS
&
GOOD COMPANY

Books I Want to Read

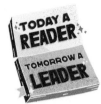

Write a list of the books you would like to read this year.

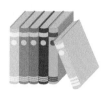

EXPAND YOUR MIND, READ A BOOK

My Favourite Films

Films can reduce stress and elicit deep feelings. They are powerful in teaching us new things and encouraging self-reflection.

Write the names of your favourite films in the tickets, then write a short review. Colour the stars to give it an overall rating.

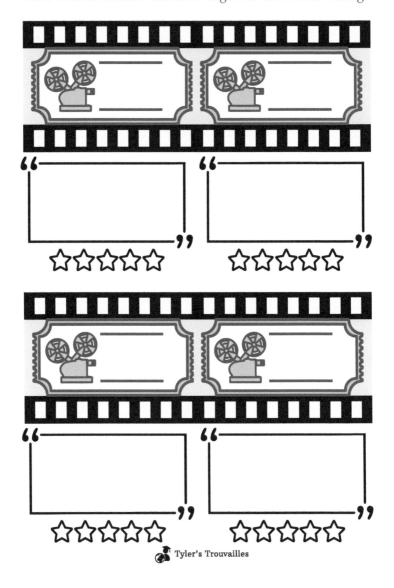

My Favourite Music

What are your favourite songs?

How do they make you feel?

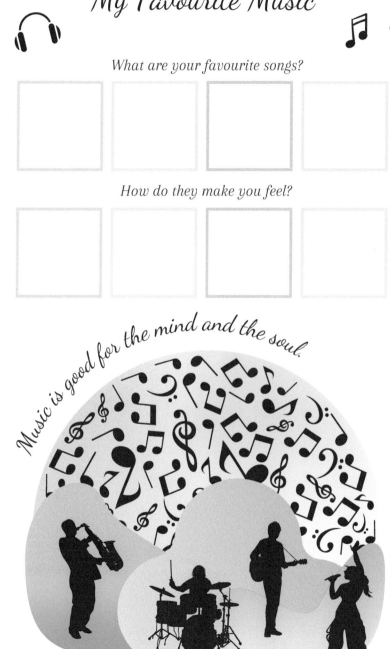

Music is good for the mind and the soul.

My Hobbies

Hobbies are interests or activities we enjoy doing in our free time. They are key for our wellbeing: relieving stress, strengthening connections and developing creativity.

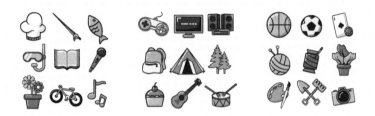

My hobbies are:

Draw pictures of yourself enjoying your hobbies.

My Habits

Habits are regular behaviours or practices
which people find difficult to give up.

Draw or write your good and bad habits in the boxes.

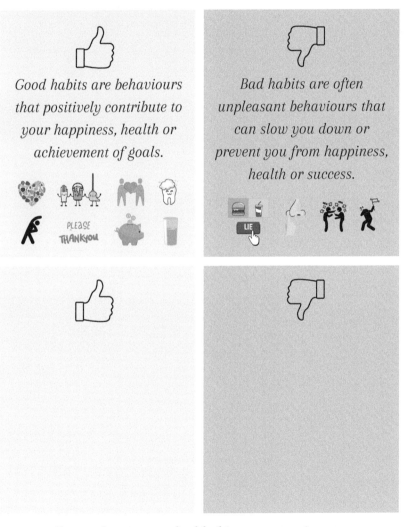

Good habits are behaviours
that positively contribute to
your happiness, health or
achievement of goals.

Bad habits are often
unpleasant behaviours that
can slow you down or
prevent you from happiness,
health or success.

*Try to change your bad habits, one at a time, to
make a positive difference to your life.*

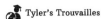 Tyler's Trouvailles

My Happy Place

Draw a place where you feel safe, happy and relaxed.
This can be a real place or from your imagination.
Use the senses boxes to add detail about your happy place.

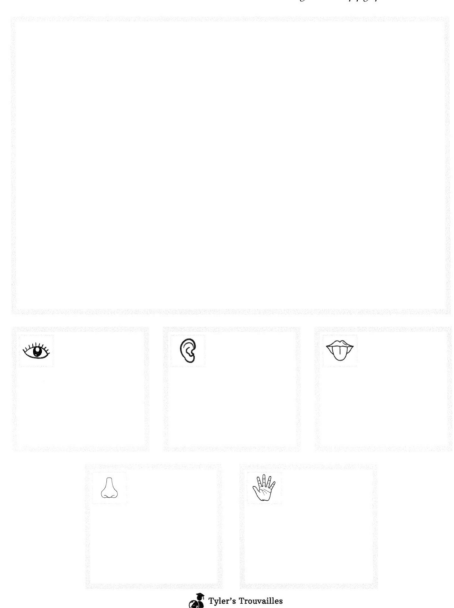

My Friends

Draw and label your friends.

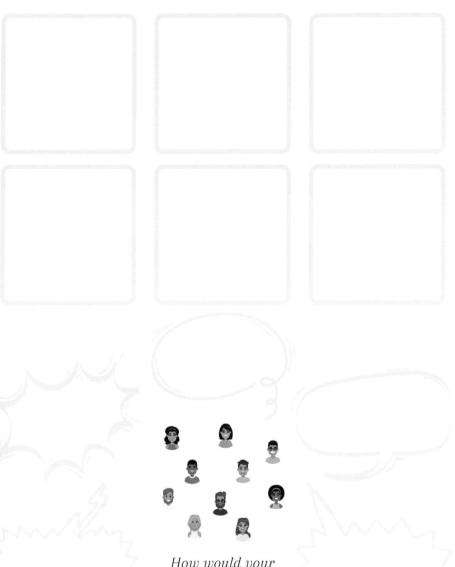

*How would your
friends describe you?*

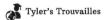 Tyler's Trouvailles

My Support Network

A support network is a group of people we can rely on and trust in times of need. They are the people we can talk to, seek advice from or will do something to help us. These people listen to us, care about us and make us feel safe.

People who may be in your support network:

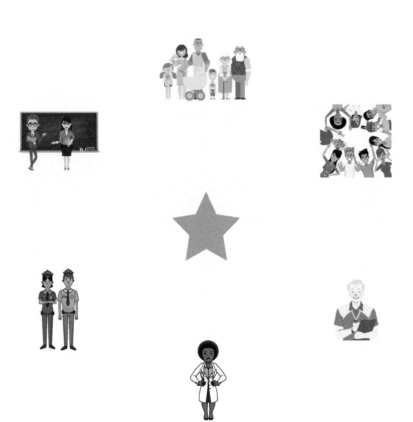

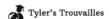

Draw around your hand. Inside your drawing, write the names of the people in your support network.

Think about the people you trust, those who you may turn to in times of need.

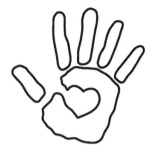

My Star Qualities

Reflect on the positive qualities you possess.
These could be your achievements, strengths, talents,
personality traits or interests.

Draw or write these in the stars-
be proud and keep shining!

I Love Me!

I love that I can...

Self-love is crucial for our wellbeing. It boosts our self-esteem, proves gratitude and motivates us to succeed.

I love that I am...

I love that I have...

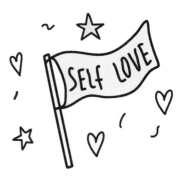

My Reflections

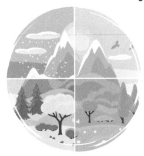

Being present and looking forward are keys to success. Nonetheless, looking back from time to time enables us to reflect on our actions, experiences and growth.

What is your best memory from last year?

What challenged you last year?

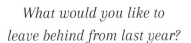

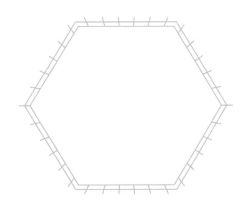

What would you like to leave behind from last year?

What did you learn about yourself last year?

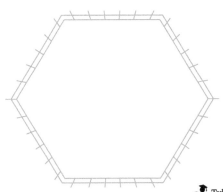

Tyler's Trouvailles

My Future

We all dream of things we want to experience, places we want to go
and things we want to achieve in our lifetime.

This is known as a bucket list.

I want to achieve...

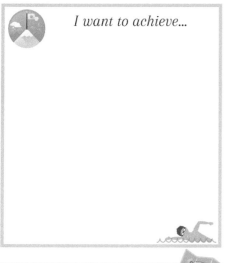

*I want to
experience...*

I want to visit...

*I want to
live in...*

because...

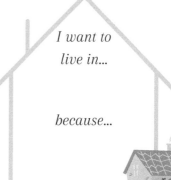

 Tyler's Trouvailles

Past Self

Reflecting on our past allows us to value our growth and consider addressing challenges we faced. Though the past cannot be changed, it gives us time to forgive, learn and motivate ourselves.

Choose an issue you had in the past or think back to a time where you experienced something significant.

Use the questions to summarise what advice you would give your past self and explain what has happened between then and now.

When did this happen?
What happened on this date?
How have you grown since then?
What should your past self be aware of?
What advice would you give to get through the challenges you faced?
How were you successful?
Who helped you along the way?
Who do you wish you had spent more time with or doing?

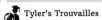 Tyler's Trouvailles

Now write these reflections in the form of a letter.

Dear Past Self,

> Writing letters can free many emotions and increase your self-awareness.

Future Self

Envisioning our future helps us focus on who we want to be and promotes goal-setting to accomplish our dreams. Though we cannot predict exactly what will happen in the future, we can make changes to ensure we are heading in the right direction.

Choose a date in the future- five years from now is ideal.
Use the questions to summarise your aspirations for the future.
This will be valuable in assessing your current direction, predicting
your future and setting goals to help make it happen.

Who and where do you want to be?
What do you want to have achieved?
Who do you want to be with?
What skills and hobbies do you want to develop?
What new friendships do you want to make?
Which new places do you want to discover?
What values will you hold?
What personal qualities do you want to develop?

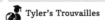

Now write these reflections in the form of a letter.

Dear Future Self,

> *Writing letters challenges thoughts about who you are, who you were and who you want to be.*

My Achievements

Reaching our goals fills us with pride and accomplishment, this defines an achievement. Achievements can be big and small, they all prove the success of something as a result of our effort, skill and courage.

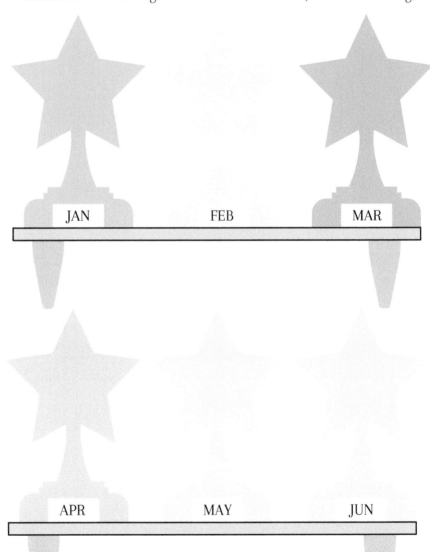

JAN   FEB   MAR

APR   MAY   JUN

Celebrate your success.

*Write your greatest achievement for each
month of the year in the star trophies.*

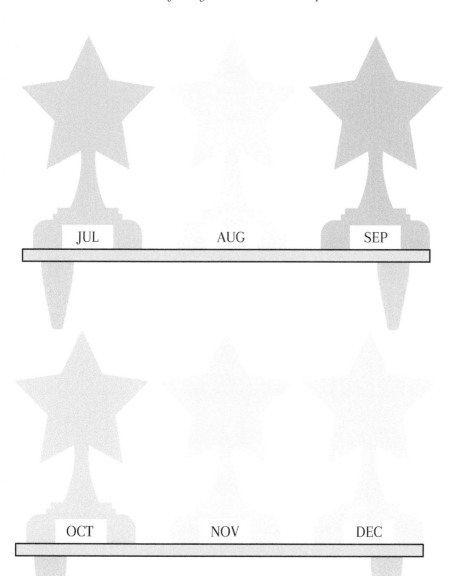

JUL   AUG   SEP

OCT   NOV   DEC

My Scrapbook

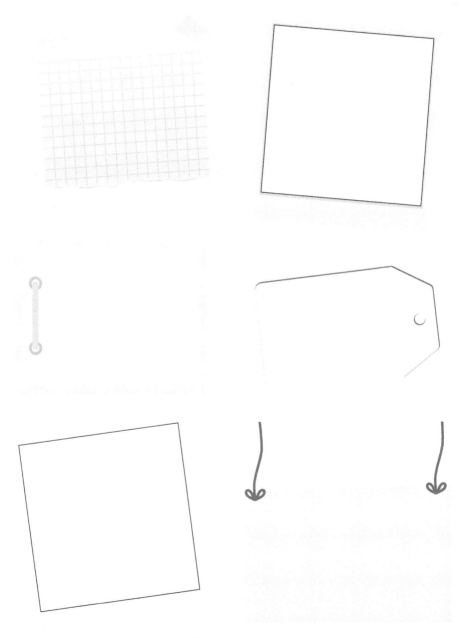

Use this as your personal scrapbook to collate your favourite memories of this year.

Compliment Calendar

Here are 52 boxes, one for each week of the year.
Compliment at least one person each week to make them feel good,
encourage them or show your appreciation.

In the boxes, you could write their name, the compliment or draw their
reaction.

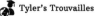

Compliments spread positivity and make others want to be around you.

Write some compliments you have received in here.

Feelings & Emotions

My Year in Colour

Colour the date to reflect how you feel about today.

Amazing Day Good Day Okay Day Bad Day Worst Day

JAN
| 1 | 2 | 3 | 4 | 5 | 6 | 7 | 8 | 9 | 10 | 11 | 12 | 13 | 14 | 15 | 16 |
| 17 | 18 | 19 | 20 | 21 | 22 | 23 | 24 | 25 | 26 | 27 | 28 | 29 | 30 | 31 |

FEB
| 1 | 2 | 3 | 4 | 5 | 6 | 7 | 8 | 9 | 10 | 11 | 12 | 13 | 14 | 15 | 16 |
| 17 | 18 | 19 | 20 | 21 | 22 | 23 | 24 | 25 | 26 | 27 | 28 | 29 |

MAR
| 1 | 2 | 3 | 4 | 5 | 6 | 7 | 8 | 9 | 10 | 11 | 12 | 13 | 14 | 15 | 16 |
| 17 | 18 | 19 | 20 | 21 | 22 | 23 | 24 | 25 | 26 | 27 | 28 | 29 | 30 | 31 |

APR
| 1 | 2 | 3 | 4 | 5 | 6 | 7 | 8 | 9 | 10 | 11 | 12 | 13 | 14 | 15 | 16 |
| 17 | 18 | 19 | 20 | 21 | 22 | 23 | 24 | 25 | 26 | 27 | 28 | 29 | 30 |

MAY
| 1 | 2 | 3 | 4 | 5 | 6 | 7 | 8 | 9 | 10 | 11 | 12 | 13 | 14 | 15 | 16 |
| 17 | 18 | 19 | 20 | 21 | 22 | 23 | 24 | 25 | 26 | 27 | 28 | 29 | 30 | 31 |

JUN
| 1 | 2 | 3 | 4 | 5 | 6 | 7 | 8 | 9 | 10 | 11 | 12 | 13 | 14 | 15 | 16 |
| 17 | 18 | 19 | 20 | 21 | 22 | 23 | 24 | 25 | 26 | 27 | 28 | 29 | 30 |

JUL
| 1 | 2 | 3 | 4 | 5 | 6 | 7 | 8 | 9 | 10 | 11 | 12 | 13 | 14 | 15 | 16 |
| 17 | 18 | 19 | 20 | 21 | 22 | 23 | 24 | 25 | 26 | 27 | 28 | 29 | 30 | 31 |

AUG
| 1 | 2 | 3 | 4 | 5 | 6 | 7 | 8 | 9 | 10 | 11 | 12 | 13 | 14 | 15 | 16 |
| 17 | 18 | 19 | 20 | 21 | 22 | 23 | 24 | 25 | 26 | 27 | 28 | 29 | 30 | 31 |

SEP
| 1 | 2 | 3 | 4 | 5 | 6 | 7 | 8 | 9 | 10 | 11 | 12 | 13 | 14 | 15 | 16 |
| 17 | 18 | 19 | 20 | 21 | 22 | 23 | 24 | 25 | 26 | 27 | 28 | 29 | 30 |

OCT
| 1 | 2 | 3 | 4 | 5 | 6 | 7 | 8 | 9 | 10 | 11 | 12 | 13 | 14 | 15 | 16 |
| 17 | 18 | 19 | 20 | 21 | 22 | 23 | 24 | 25 | 26 | 27 | 28 | 29 | 30 | 31 |

NOV
| 1 | 2 | 3 | 4 | 5 | 6 | 7 | 8 | 9 | 10 | 11 | 12 | 13 | 14 | 15 | 16 |
| 17 | 18 | 19 | 20 | 21 | 22 | 23 | 24 | 25 | 26 | 27 | 28 | 29 | 30 |

DEC
| 1 | 2 | 3 | 4 | 5 | 6 | 7 | 8 | 9 | 10 | 11 | 12 | 13 | 14 | 15 | 16 |
| 17 | 18 | 19 | 20 | 21 | 22 | 23 | 24 | 25 | 26 | 27 | 28 | 29 | 30 | 31 |

Emotions, Feelings & Mood

These words are often used interchangeably- in a way where many of us believe emotions, feelings and mood mean the same thing. Put simply, the main difference is time.

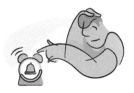

Emotions

- Brain to body chemical messages that help us understand our environment

- Temporary and intense

- Automatic and universally expressed

- Triggers are easily identifiable

Feelings

- Low-key but sustainable

- Requires cognitive awareness

- Fuelled by a mix of emotions

- Connects, reflects and are shaped by personal experiences and reasoning

Mood

- Long-term, often days

- Gradual onset

- Generalised-difficult to identify specific triggers

- Complex-influenced by our mental state, physiology and environment

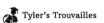

*Use the clouds to draw expressions that reflect
feelings and emotions you have experienced.*

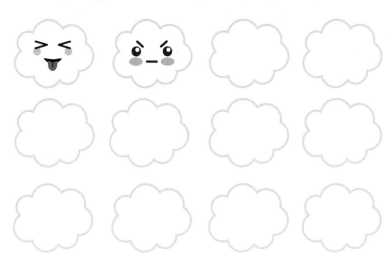

*Use this space to draw or write about your
current feelings or mood.
Think about your most recent emotions.*

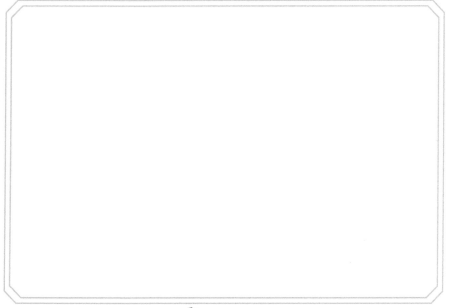

Thoughts, Feelings & Behaviours

Our thoughts, feelings and behaviours are all connected. Our thoughts lead to a feeling that results in reactive behaviours. It is important to recognise this relationship and consider changing our thought processes to promote positive feelings and actions.

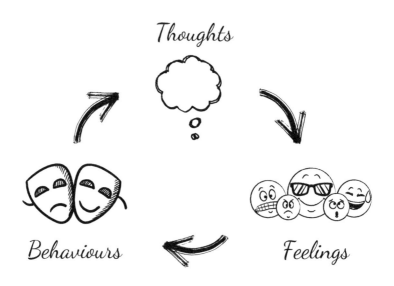

Thoughts

Behaviours

Feelings

Thoughts describe an idea, image, opinion or belief produced by thinking. They often exist as words in our minds which reflect what we are experiencing.	Feelings are closely related to our emotions. These come and go depending on what we are experiencing. Often, we experience many feelings each day.	Behaviours define how we act: the things we do and the way we behave. Many factors can influence our behaviours- the importance is to have control.

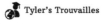 Tyler's Trouvailles

Not all thoughts are true. They can sometimes be guesses or a product of overthinking. It is essential to remember what we can and cannot control, whilst considering new, positive thoughts to help us see a situation differently. This will influence our feelings and behaviours.

Reflect...

Think back to a time where you reacted too quickly or overthought something. What happened?

Describe your thoughts, feelings and behaviours during this situation.

Now, choose a new thought. What might have changed as a result?

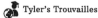 Tyler's Trouvailles

Emotional Awareness

Emotional awareness is the ability to recognise and understand our own emotions and feelings, as well as those of others. Emotions are complex and can be influenced by many things. All emotions are necessary for a healthy life.

Imagine each of these beans are a different emotion. The beans represent growth- growth in emotional maturity and our ability to thrive, even when we experience strong emotions.
How many different emotions can you think of?
Write them in the beans.

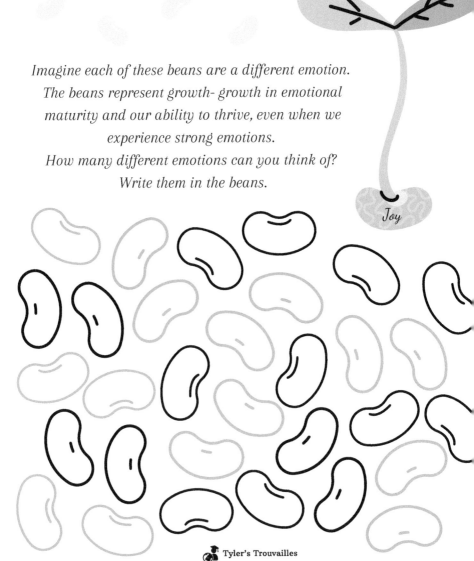

Joy

How do you feel?

Emotion and Feeling:

Why do you feel this way? How do you know?

How does your friend feel?

Emotion and Feeling:

Why do they feel this way? How do you know?

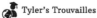

Emotions Tree

As humans, we experience many emotions during our lives. There are six basic, universally recognisable emotions: anger, joy, fear, disgust, sadness and surprise. Complex emotions can combine multiple basic emotions or are rooted in them. Our emotions can affect our behaviour in different ways and are often temporary.

Each branch represents a basic emotion.
Add leaves to these branches with other associated emotions and feelings rooted in them.

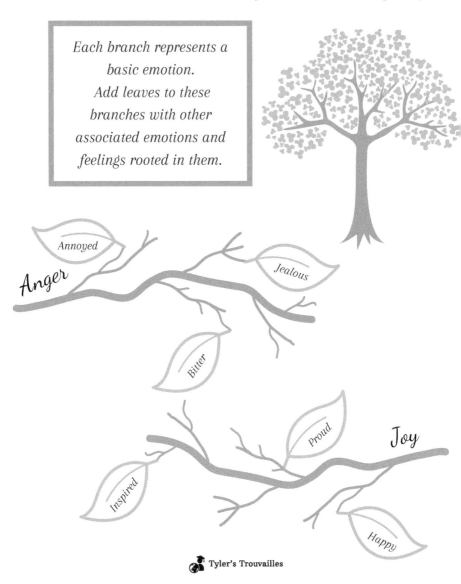

Anger

Annoyed

Jealous

Bitter

Proud

Joy

Inspired

Happy

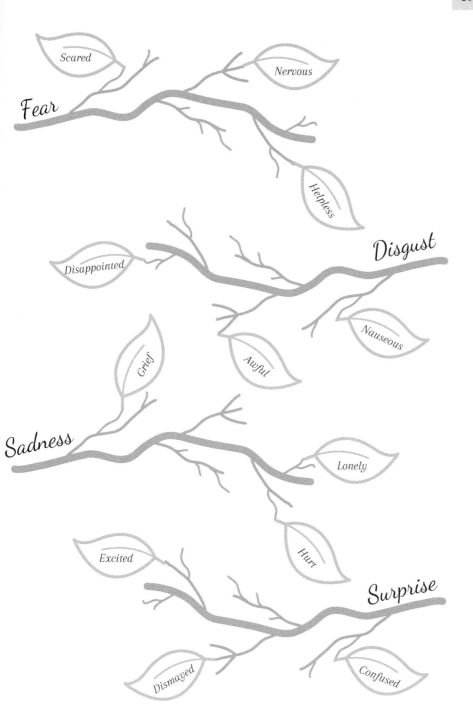

Colours and Emotions

Colours and emotions are closely linked, meaning some colours can influence our mood or emotions. Our feelings about colour are often personal and rooted in our own experience or culture.

*Write the feelings and emotions **you** associate with each colour.*

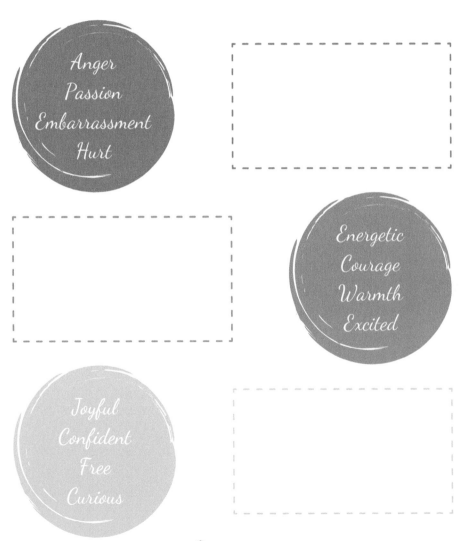

Anger
Passion
Embarrassment
Hurt

Energetic
Courage
Warmth
Excited

Joyful
Confident
Free
Curious

Disgust
Disappointed
Calm
Growth

Sad
Peaceful
Sleepy
Patient

Fearful
Wise
Mysterious
Strength

Powerful
Bored
Miserable
Lonely

Recognising Feelings & Emotions

Recognising and understanding our feelings and emotions is vital for our wellbeing. It is important to talk about how we feel so we are able to manage our feelings effectively.

Mood Mountain

Where are you on Mood Mountain today?
Talk to your family and peers, where are they on Mood Mountain?
Reflect and discuss your feelings.

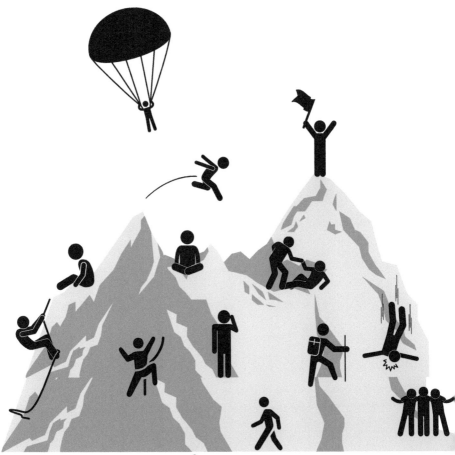

Use this table to record some key feelings you or someone you know has experienced this year. What feeling or emotion have you/they experienced? Who experienced it? When was this? Why do you/they feel this way?

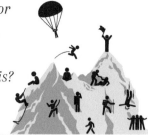

Proud	Me 20.07.2022	My handwriting has improved a lot this year.

My Experience with:
Anger

What things do you say?

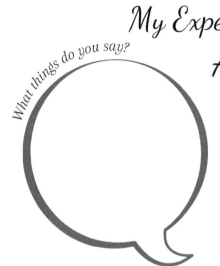

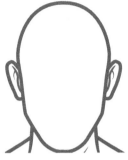

What does your face look like when you are angry?

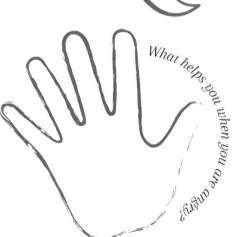

What helps you when you are angry?

How do you behave?

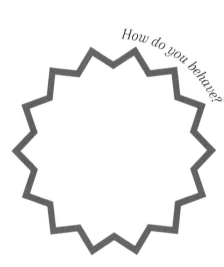

What do you know about anger?

What happens to your body?

 Tyler's Trouvailles

What pushes my buttons?

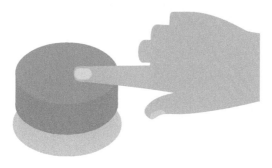

Write in the buttons some situations or things that make you angry.

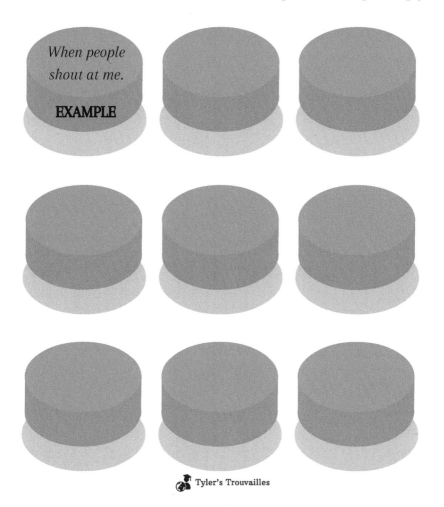

When people shout at me.

EXAMPLE

My Experience with:
Sadness

What things do you say?

What does your face look like when you are sad?

How do you behave?

What helps you when you are sad?

What do you know about sadness?

What happens to your body?

Sadness

Draw or write the things that make you feel sad.

Feeling blue... what could you do?

Talk to someone in
your support network.

Cry. It is okay to cry.
Take slow, deep breaths.

Listen to your
favourite music.

Go for a walk outside
and reflect.

Do something you
enjoy.

Ask for a hug.

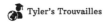 Tyler's Trouvailles

My Experience with:
Joy

What things do you say?

What does your face look like when you are joyful?

How do you behave?

What helps you stay joyful?

What do you know about joy?

What happens to your body?

What makes me happy?

Consider who, when, where and what makes you happy.

Why do these things make you happy?

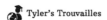

My Experience with:
Fear

What things do you say?

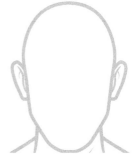

What does your face look like when you are fearful?

What helps you when you are scared?

How do you behave?

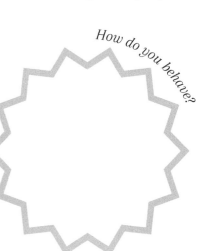

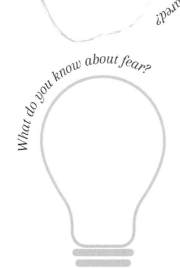

What do you know about fear?

What happens to your body?

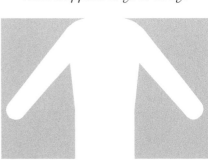

 Tyler's Trouvailles

Fear Factor

Everyone has fears. Some fears are bigger than others.
Organise your fears by writing or drawing whether they are small,
moderate or extreme fears.

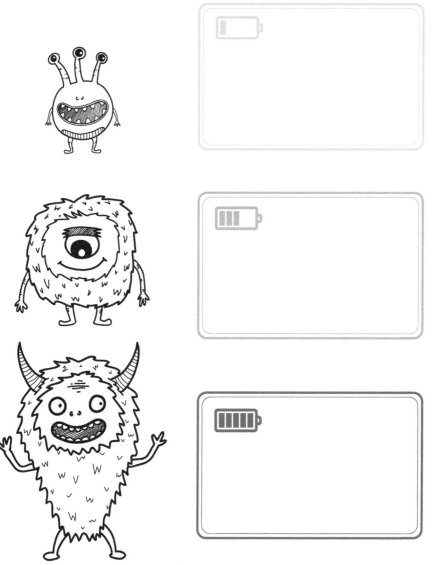

My Experience with:
Disgust

What things do you say?

What does your face look like when you are disgusted?

How do you behave?

What helps you when you feel disgusted?

What do you know about disgust?

What happens to your body?

Disgust

Draw or write the things that make you feel disgusted.

*Fill the circles with
memories of times
when you felt
disgusted.*

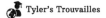

My Experience with:
Surprise

What things do you say?

What does your face look like when you are surprised?

How do you behave?

What helps you when you feel surprised?

What do you know about surprise?

What happens to your body?

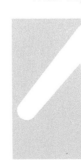
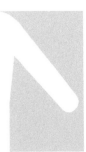

Surprise

Being surprised by something can cause us to feel comfortable or uncomfortable- sometimes both at the same time.

Draw or write examples of these in the boxes.

Comfortable

Uncomfortable

A surprise I would like:

A surprise my family would like:

A surprise my friend would like:

A surprise my teacher would like:

Control

In life, we often stress or worry about things we cannot control. This can make us lose focus on the things we can control, therefore impacting our feelings and experiences. It is important to remember this, especially when times are tough.

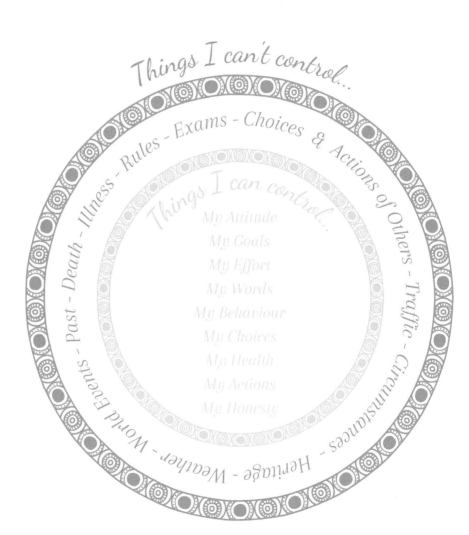

Things I can't control...

Illness - Rules - Exams - Choices & Actions of Others - Traffic - Circumstances - Heritage - Weather - World Events - Past - Death

Things I can control...

My Attitude
My Goals
My Effort
My Words
My Behaviour
My Choices
My Health
My Actions
My Honesty

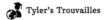

Things I can work on:

Things I cannot control or change:

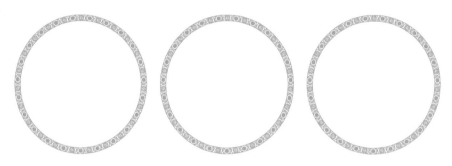

Strategies to help me...

 Write a journal

 Take time to think & accept

 Set goals & targets

 Break it down or create a schedule

 Talk to someone or ask for help

 Be kind to yourself

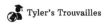

Tyler's Trouvailles

Anxiety

Anxiety is the feeling of unease, worry, dread or fear. It is a survival response and in small doses, it is healthy and good for us. We usually feel anxious about things that are going to happen or things we think might happen in the future.

What makes you anxious?
Which situations make you feel uncomfortable?

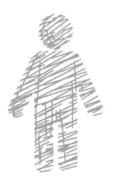

What negative thoughts do you have in these situations?

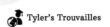

What is your experience with worry? How does your body respond? Circle or add your own.

 Dizzy

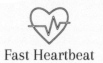 Fast Heartbeat

 Headache

 Blushing

Uncomfortable

 Emotional

Aches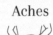

Confused

 Quiet

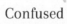

Coping Strategies

Self-Talk

What things could you do to calm your emotions?

 Meditate

 Read

 Exercise

Draw

How could I prepare myself?

How have I managed this before?

What is in my control?

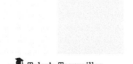

Worry Bottles

Worries are negative thoughts. We worry about things from the past or the future, often things that have not even happened.

We all have worries- some small worries and some much bigger.

Some worries can be helpful as they can guide our problem-solving skills and productivity.

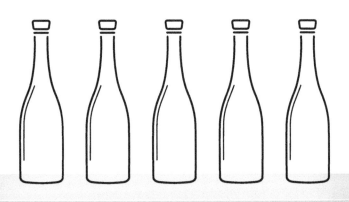

Fill the small bottles with smaller, everyday worries and the bigger bottles with the things you worry about the most.

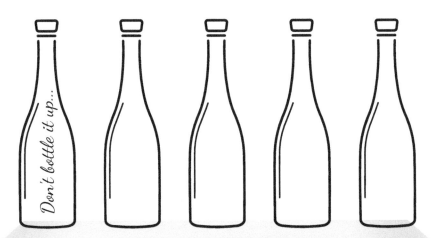

Don't bottle it up...

Worries

Work on emptying your worry bottles.
Focus on those that need the most attention.
It is always better to talk about your worries
to make them more manageable.
Remember- you are not alone.

Write and draw your four favourite, trusted adults that make
you feel safe and are always there to listen to you.

Fight, Flight or Freeze?

Fight-flight-freeze responses are our body's natural, automatic reactions to danger and trauma. Worries can also trigger a response of fight, flight or freeze. This is what causes us to feel anxious.

Fight

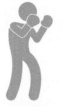

- Feeling a rush of energy and tense muscles
- Angry, irritable, aggressive
- Using unkind words
- Physical e.g. hitting, kicking, throwing, biting
- Screaming and shouting
- Defensive and blaming others
- Moving towards the threat

Flight

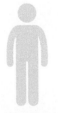

- Feeling a burst of energy to run or escape
- Anxious, overwhelmed, panicked
- Fidgety and hyperactive
- Struggling to focus and concentrate
- Avoiding or ignoring the situation
- Shallow breathing
- Moving away from the threat

Freeze

- Feeling stuck and unresponsive
- Numb, helpless, depressed
- Disengaged, withdrawn or daydreaming
- Unable to move your body
- Refusing or not knowing how to answer
- Difficulty making decisions
- Wanting to hide or isolate yourself

Fight-flight-freeze is caused by a hormone in our bodies called adrenaline that is released when we feel strong emotions. We often experience different reactions depending on the scenario. This can be a result of our previous experiences and feelings of similar situations or the uncertainty of something new.

Name a situation that makes you worry or you see as a threat: *Circle your response.*   *How does/did it make you feel and why?*

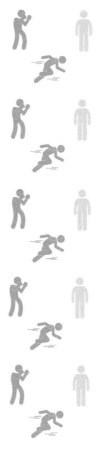

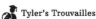

Grief & Loss

Grief is a strong, natural reaction we experience when we lose something or someone close to us. There are many stages to grief, including: denial, anger, bargaining, depression and acceptance. Each stage presents different emotions, for different lengths of time.

Who or what are you grieving?

How do you feel? How does your body feel?

How will your life be different now?

Which stage of grief are you experiencing now?

Denial
"Is this really happening?"

What helps you to cope with this feeling?

Anger
"Why is this happening to me?"

Bargaining
"I will do anything to change this."

What do you need from your family, friends and others now?

Depression
"What is the point of life now?"

Acceptance
"It's going to be okay."

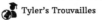 Tyler's Trouvailles

Though it can be difficult to think positively when experiencing grief and loss, it is important to connect to positive feelings.

Fill the hearts from the memory box with happy thoughts and memories that remind you of who or what you have lost- treasure these moments.

I wish...

_ _ _ _ _ _ _ _ _ _ _

_ _ _ _ _ _ _ _ _ _

_ _ _ _ _ _ _ _ _ _

_ _ _ _ _ _ _ _ _ _ _

_ _ _ _ _ _ _ _ _ _ _

What questions do you have about this loss?

MEMORIES

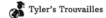 Tyler's Trouvailles

Change

Change describes an act, event or process through which something becomes different. It can be challenging, but it can also be transforming: developing our resilience, confidence and understanding of the world and ourselves. Change sparks many different feelings and emotions- these can change over time and range in intensity.

Draw some emotions you may experience during change.

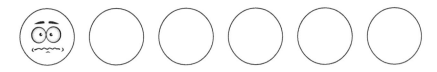

Write or draw some examples of expected and unexpected changes.

Some changes are expected- these we can prepare for.

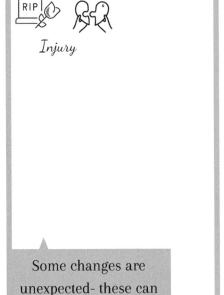

Injury

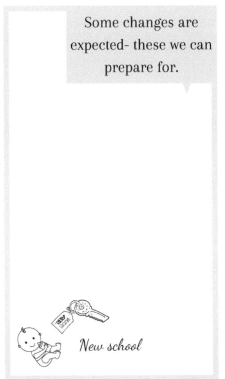

New school

Some changes are unexpected- these can surprise us and can be more challenging.

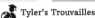 Tyler's Trouvailles

Changes come in different sizes and forms. They can impact our lives in many different ways. Sometimes, even the smallest things can be life-changing.

Coping Strategies:

- Prepare, where possible
- Talk about your feelings
- Read and talk about changes
- Be kind to yourself

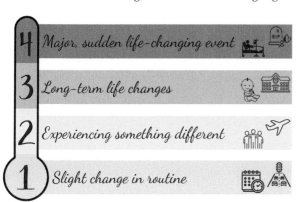

4 | Major, sudden life-changing event
3 | Long-term life changes
2 | Experiencing something different
1 | Slight change in routine

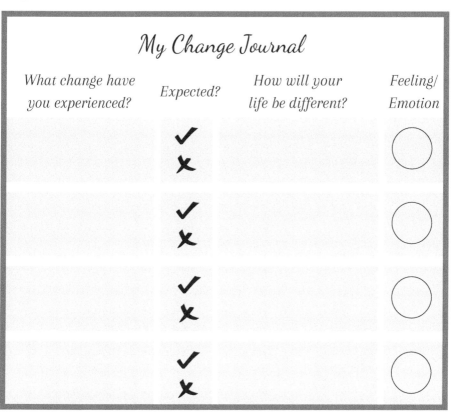

My Change Journal

What change have you experienced?	Expected?	How will your life be different?	Feeling/ Emotion
	✔ ✘		◯
	✔ ✘		◯
	✔ ✘		◯
	✔ ✘		◯

Managing Difficult Emotions

Difficult emotions can make us feel upset and uncomfortable. They often make us feel out of control and can be a result of many different things. Managing emotions is healthy- it means choosing how and when to express the emotions we feel.

When might you experience a difficult emotion?

Recognise

Recognise, describe and name the emotion or feeling you are experiencing.

Allow & Accept

Allow and accept it, even if it is uncomfortable or unwelcome.

Investigate

Investigate where and why you are experiencing this emotion or feeling.

Nurture

Take care of yourself. This does not define you, it will pass, it is temporary.

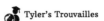

Tyler's Trouvailles

Make notes as you experience this 'RAIN'.

 Feelings Forecast

Control your emotions, don't let them control you.

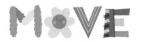 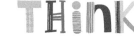

Talk to others about your feelings. Ask for advice.

Move your body to make you feel better. Walk, run, dance...

Think about positive, funny or happy memories.

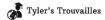 Tyler's Trouvailles

My Best and My Worst

We all have good and bad days. Our sense of self-worth can vary depending on where we are, who we are with, what is happening and our reaction to different situations. It is important to reflect on these times and experiences to help us learn, grow and surround ourselves with the kindness we deserve.

When do you feel your best?

When do you feel your worst?

Where do you feel your best?

Where do you feel your worst?

Who makes you feel amazing?

Who brings you down?

When was the best day of your life?

When was the worst day of your life

What emotions did you experience?

What emotions did you experience?

My Words

Sometimes our words can hurt the feelings of others, sometimes even ourselves. It is important that we take time to reflect before we speak.

If you're feeling snappy... STOP & THINK.
Are my words...

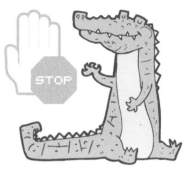

TRUE?

HELPFUL?

INSPIRING?

NECESSARY?

KIND?

Reflect on a time when you said something to someone that hurt their feelings. Make notes on your thoughts at the time, what you said and what you could say next time.

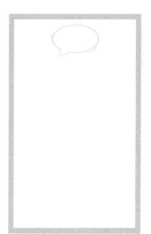

Saying Sorry

Saying sorry can be difficult for us to do. Sometimes, quite the opposite, we say it too quickly without any meaning or understanding for why we are apologising.

Apologising allows us to communicate- expressing our regret and showing we care about the feelings and perspectives of others.

When might you need to say sorry to someone?

Remember to be calm and sincere when you say sorry.

Take deep breaths and use this script to help you make a genuine apology.

I am sorry for...

It was wrong because...

Next time I will...

How can I make it better?

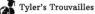 Tyler's Trouvailles

Admitting you have made a mistake can take a lot bravery.

Draw or write about a time you apologised for something you did. How did you feel? How did they feel? How would you act next time?

Fill in the script to create a meaningful apology for what you did.

I am sorry for...

It was wrong because...

Next time I will...

How can I make it better?

Speaking Openly

Saying 'no' can be challenging for many reasons.
We often say 'yes' to avoid hurting the feelings of others, but in the process we can hurt ourselves.

Fill the boxes with different ways of saying 'no'.

Saying 'no' with kindness...

Thank you for thinking of me, but I can't, I am busy.

For example, when you do not want to join in with an activity, want your opinion to be heard or when you are busy.

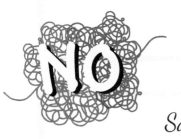

Saying 'no' firmly...

Stop! I don't like that, it hurts.

For example, when someone is hurting you, forcing you to do something unsafe or making you feel uncomfortable.

How to say difficult things with kindness...

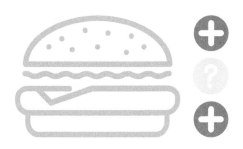

Sometimes our opinions may not be what others want to hear. It is important we do not lie and stay true to ourselves, whilst also being mindful of their feelings.

A good way to do this would be to construct it like a burger or a sandwich. Share feedback or say the difficult, more sensitive part of our opinion in the middle (filling) of two positive things (the bread).

Reflect on a time when you had to say something difficult to someone. Try making a kindness burger to share your honesty.

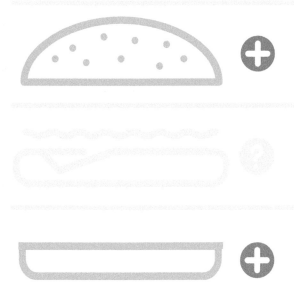

Self-Esteem

Self-esteem defines our overall opinions of ourselves- what we think, feel and believe about our own abilities and limitations.

Colour the stars to show how much you believe and agree with each statement.

1 star = you disagree and do not believe it.
5 stars = you completely agree and strongly believe it.

I love who I am ☆☆☆☆☆

I believe in myself ☆☆☆☆☆

I am important ☆☆☆☆☆

I like the way I look ☆☆☆☆☆

I know my positive qualities ☆☆☆☆☆

I like trying new things ☆☆☆☆☆

I respect myself ☆☆☆☆☆

I am resilient ☆☆☆☆☆

I work well with others ☆☆☆☆☆

I aim to challenge myself ☆☆☆☆☆

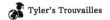 Tyler's Trouvailles

Overall, how would you rate your self-esteem?

☆☆☆☆☆

How could you boost your self-esteem?

take care of your mind

☐ Be kind and have a positive attitude.

☐ Do not compare yourself to others.

☐ Accept who you are, including your flaws!

☐ Celebrate the small stuff...and the big!

Self-Worth

Self-worth is the internal recognition that we are valuable as individuals: worthy of belonging and love from others.

Signs of Low Self-Worth

- Disliking and being unkind to yourself
- Negatively comparing yourself to others
- Believing others are better than you
- Changing or lying about yourself because you are desperate to fit in
- Being harsh on yourself when you make a mistake
- Not accepting compliments
- Seeing the world as a negative place
- Feeling uncomfortable alone and with others

Signs of High Self-Worth

- Believing in yourself
- Confidence and optimism
- Enjoying time alone and with others
- Seeing the world as a friendly, positive place to learn and grow
- Respecting differences in yourself and others
- Accepting of mistakes and learning from them
- Encouraging others
- Embracing change and challenge
- Expressing yourself through effective communication

What actions are you taking to boost your self-worth?

Below is a list of general feeling statements.
Draw an arrow on the scale to show how strongly you
disagree (0) or agree (12) with each statement.

I feel that I am worthy, as worthy as everyone.

I feel that I have lots of good qualities.

I feel that I am not succeeding.

I am able to do things as well as most other people.

I feel I do not have much to be proud of.

I have a positive attitude towards myself.

I wish I could be like others or change myself.

I wish I could have more respect for myself.

Talk to a trusted adult to reflect on your self-evaluation.

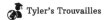 Tyler's Trouvailles

Positive Affirmations

Positive affirmations describe positive statements that help us challenge and overcome negative thoughts or beliefs. Repeating these often and genuinely believing them helps us to make positive changes to our thoughts, feelings and our self-esteem.

I am kind.

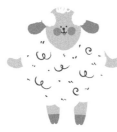

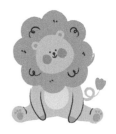

I am brave.

I can make a difference.

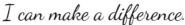

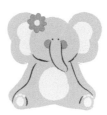

I am loved.

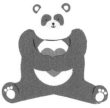

I can do this.

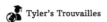

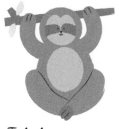

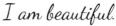

Write your own positive affirmations in the stars.

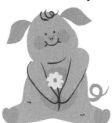

I believe in me.

I can do anything.

I matter.

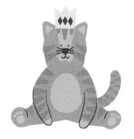

I am amazing.

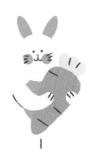

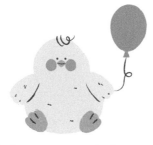

I deserve good things.

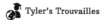 Tyler's Trouvailles

Life Skills, Values & Personal Qualities

Acceptance

Acceptance is the process of accepting someone or something. It is about learning to be at peace and creating positive relationships with ourselves, our differences and experiences.

Draw or write the things you accept and love about yourself.

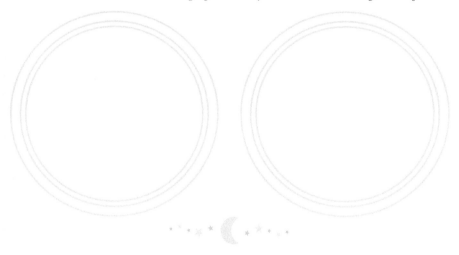

In life, we all make mistakes. The important thing to remember is that we must accept these mistakes and learn from the lessons they teach us.

Mistakes...   *Lessons...*

Accountability

Accountability defines being committed and willing to take responsibility for our actions and decisions.
It proves our dedication to creating a positive impact, therefore can boost our productivity and performance.

SEE IT

OWN IT

SOLVE IT

DO IT

List three ways you could show accountability in your daily life.

When have you shown accountability at home or at school?

How did it make you feel?

How did it make others feel?

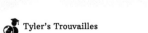 Tyler's Trouvailles

Adaptability

Being adaptable means being open-minded and flexible to change.
Adaptability encourages acceptance through promoting new skills and
positive behaviours to react efficiently to changing circumstances.

In life, there are many events and situations where
we may need to adapt. Some examples include:

- Birth of a new sibling
- Moving house or school
- Changing classes
- Illness

- Change in routine
- Family separation
- Loss
- Unexpected events

Identify a situation where you had to adapt:

Explain how you adapted to this change:

Why was it important for you to adapt?

Ambition

Being ambitious means we strive to achieve our desires and accomplish our goals. Ambition is our drive to succeed- it keeps us focused on our hopes, goals and dreams.

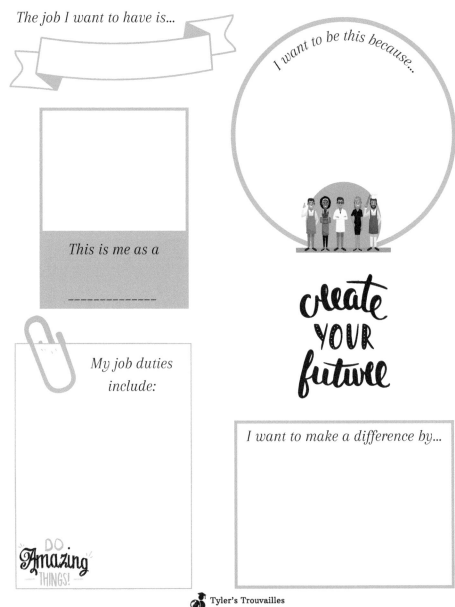

The job I want to have is...

I want to be this because...

This is me as a

_____

My job duties include:

DO Amazing THINGS!

create YOUR future

I want to make a difference by...

Appreciation

Appreciation is the recognition, understanding and enjoyment of the good qualities of someone or something. It involves being grateful for the beauty and excellence they hold- this can motivate us and put things into perspective.

Draw or write the people, places and things you appreciate in your life.

PEOPLE

PLACES

THINGS

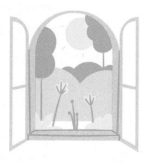

Awareness

Awareness is the knowledge and understanding that something is happening or exists: self, social and environmental. It involves recognising different perspectives and highlights that all of our choices have consequences. Awareness helps us feel grounded, boosts our confidence and supports us to become more efficient.

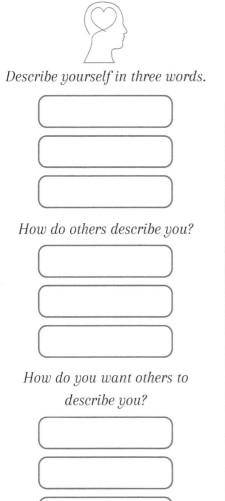

Describe yourself in three words.

How do others describe you?

How do you want others to describe you?

Write some of the key themes or headlines in the news today or this week.

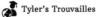

Tyler's Trouvailles

Balance

Work-life or school-life balance is the positive relationship and time dedicated to working, as well as the important things in our lives like family, hobbies, socialising, volunteering, etc. Balance is crucial for a healthy, happy life, as it allows us to focus but also reduces stress.

It is easier to find your balance by separating your needs and responsibilities with your wants and desires.

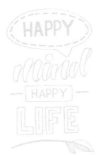

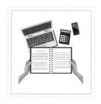
Draw or write the different things that form balanced living for you.
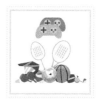

Calm

Being calm involves controlling our feelings and strong emotions by not always showing them or allowing them to control us.

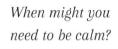

When might you need to be calm?

Staying calm gives your mind clarity, meaning you are able to think clearly and make better decisions.

Calming Strategies:

- Take deep breaths
- Talk to someone
- Take a walk
- Listen to music
- Have a bath
- Enjoy a hobby
- Think positive thoughts

My Cup of Calm

Draw or write the things you could do to help you stay calm.

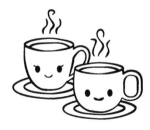

Compassion

Being compassionate means showing care and concern for others and living things, especially when they are suffering. Self-compassion is about showing this understanding and kindness to ourselves too.

Write three ways you could show care and compassion towards yourself or others.

1.

2.

3.

I showed compassion when...

Someone showed me compassion when...

Compassion reduces anxiety and stress, therefore increasing possibilities for happiness, connection and perspective.

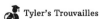 Tyler's Trouvailles

Courage

Courage is having the strength to explore new opportunities and make good choices, even when fear or obstacles try to hold us back.

I showed courage when...

Fears I have overcome through courage:

Draw two courageous people you know.

Write encouraging messages to help find your courage and bravery.

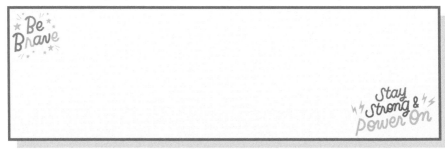

Be Brave

Stay Strong & Power On

Creativity

Creativity is about using our imagination to create something original and unique. Thinking creatively involves being open-minded to think of things from a new and different perspective.

- Pursue your passions and interests
- Reduce your screen time
- Avoid shaming, criticism and comparison
- Explore and try new things
- Find time to be creative

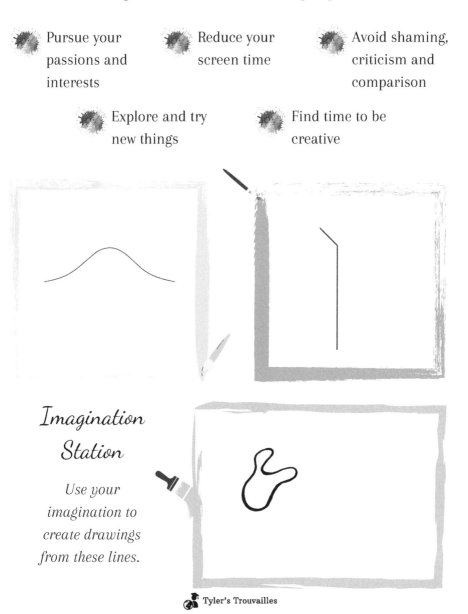

Imagination Station

Use your imagination to create drawings from these lines.

Communication

Communication defines how we give, receive and share information. We can communicate in many ways: speaking, writing, listening, reading and acting. It is fundamental for our existence and survival. Effective communication is crucial for deepening our understanding, developing positive relationships and promoting prosperity.

Ways to Communicate...

An Effective Communicator...

- Actively listens
- Respects others
- Speaks clearly and concisely

What are the benefits of effective communication?

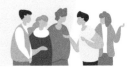

What information needs communicating? Why?

When have you communicated today? Why?

How could you improve your communication skills?

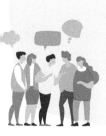

Tyler's Trouvailles

Confidence

Confidence is about feeling sure and secure about ourselves and abilities. Self-love plays an important part in boosting our confidence, self-esteem and acceptance of ourselves.

Write kind words about yourself in the hearts.

Draw or write the physical features you like about yourself.

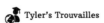 Tyler's Trouvailles

Imagine you are meeting yourself.

What kind things would you say about your talents, qualities and appearance?

> Write a list of ten kind compliments to yourself.

1.

2.

3.

> Find time to look in a real mirror and say these to yourself.

4.

5.

6.

> This will challenge negative thoughts and remind you just how amazing you are!

7.

8.

9.

10.

Connection

Connecting is the process of creating and building relationships with others. Connection is crucial for happiness, as it helps us regulate emotions, develops support networks and provides a sense of purpose.

 Why is connection important?

How can you connect with other people?

Find someone who...

Has travelled to another country:

Can play a musical instrument:

Likes the same foods as you:

Has a family member with a disability:

Has more than two siblings:

Speaks more than one language:

Is left handed:

Has a birthday in March:

Has a different nationality:

Curiosity

Curiosity defines the strong desire to know or learn something new. It is a deep interest that leads to questioning and investigation-opening up a world of infinite opportunities and discoveries.

If I wrote a book, it would be about...

If I could eat anything for the rest of my life, it would be...

If I could go anywhere, I would go...

If I could meet anyone, I would choose...

If I could have a superpower, it would be...

If I could build anything, I would build...

If I could change anything about the world, it would be...

Things I want to find out...

Determination

Determination embraces our perseverance, passion and motivation towards achieving our goals. Goals give us a clearer focus and provides control of our future. They are desired aims we are committed to achieving. They are our keys to success.

This Year I Will...

START

STOP

Try ✓

≡GO

DO :)

Top 3 Goals:

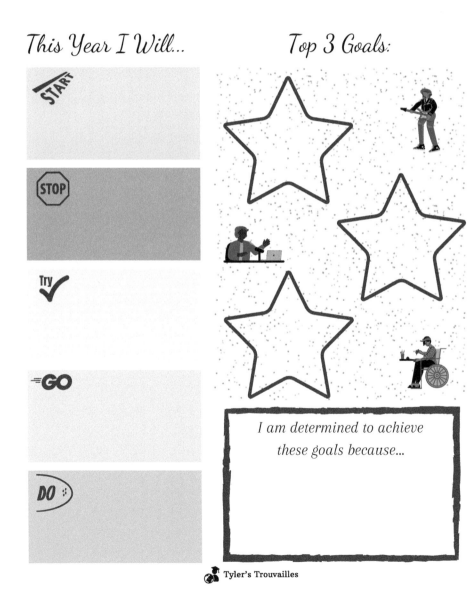

I am determined to achieve
these goals because...

Discipline

Discipline provides us with expectations and rules that often have consequences if not followed. It helps create positive habits and routines in making us effective and efficient individuals.

Different places and people have different rules you are expected to follow. Write the rules you have to follow at home and at school below.

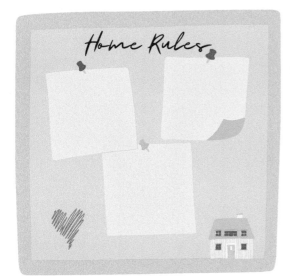

What are the consequences when you do not follow these rules?

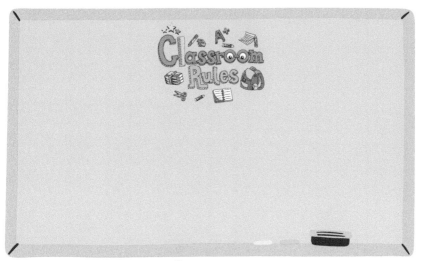

Diversity

Diversity includes the understanding and acceptance of differences, it is valuable in realising different perspectives and experiences. Our world is amazing and diverse. We are all alike, but all different at the same time. We are all unique.

Draw three friends in the polaroids, then consider what is the same and what is different about you and your friends.

Same

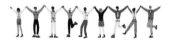

Different

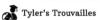

Empathy

Empathy defines our ability to understand and share the feelings of one another. It is really important in helping us communicate, regulating our own feelings and responding appropriately to different situations.

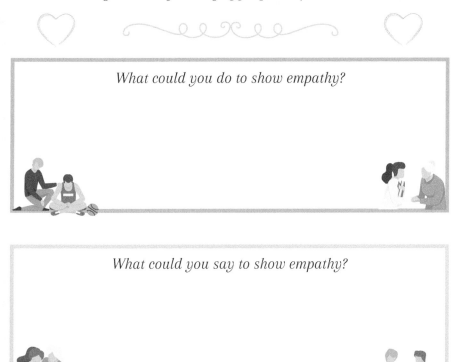

What could you do to show empathy?

What could you say to show empathy?

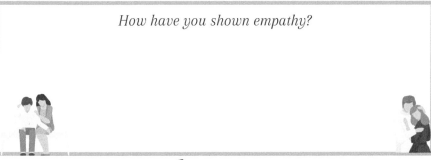

How have you shown empathy?

Equality

Equality is all about treating everybody with respect and giving everyone equal opportunities, regardless of our differences. It ensures we are all included and have the freedom to share our experiences, knowledge and skills with others.

Examples of Equality Characteristics:

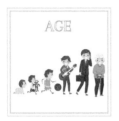
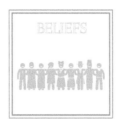
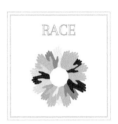

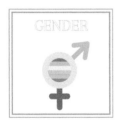
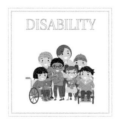
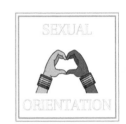

Equality promotes a society that is...

Why do you think equality is important?

Productive

Accepting

Fairness

Fairness is all about equity.

It means that every one of us must get what we need, what we deserve and what is appropriate for us as an individual, to give everyone access to the same experiences and opportunities.

How to be Fair:

- Be open-minded
- Follow rules
- Be honest
- Be responsible for your choices and mistakes
- Share and take turns
- Be kind
- _____
- _____

How have you shown fairness to others?

How does it feel when you are treated unfairly?

Forgiveness

Forgiveness is when you choose to let go and choose peace, even when you have been hurt by someone or something. It is not about revenge, but instead, focusing on your own happiness and growth.

When have you shown forgiveness?

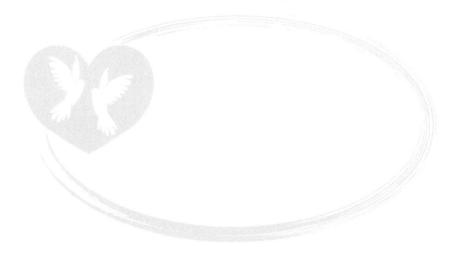

What emotions have you experienced during the process of forgiveness?

When has someone forgiven you?

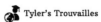 Tyler's Trouvailles

Freedom

Freedom defines our power, ability and right to act, speak and think as we choose. This enables us to pursue happiness and express individuality.

What does freedom mean to you?

A song that reminds you of freedom...

How do you experience freedom?

An image that reminds you of freedom...

In what ways do you lack freedom?

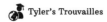 Tyler's Trouvailles

Friendship

Friendships are positive relationships between people. They are built on mutual trust, affection and support. True friends have our best interests at heart, providing us with a sense of belonging and purpose through both good times and bad times.

A Good Friend...

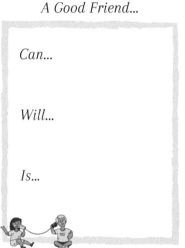

Can...

Will...

Is...

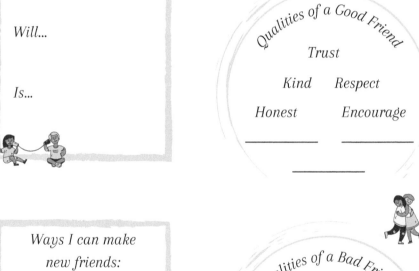

Qualities of a Good Friend

Trust

Kind   *Respect*

Honest   *Encourage*

_____   _____

_____

Ways I can make new friends:

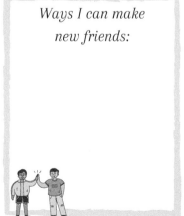

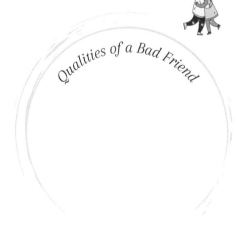

Qualities of a Bad Friend

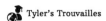

friends

Choose three friends and draw them in the polaroids.
In the boxes, draw or write what makes them a good
friend to you and the activities you enjoy doing together.

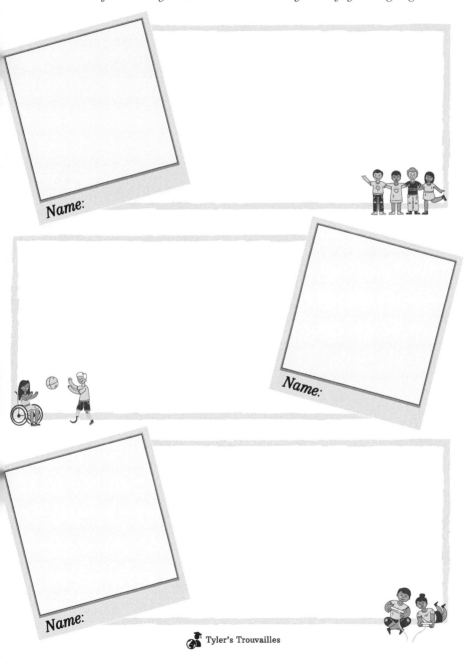

Name:

Name:

Name:

Tyler's Trouvailles

Giving

Giving is the act of transferring something we have to benefit, support and make a difference to something or someone else. It is a generous and meaningful way to show we care, leading to greater happiness for both the giver and the recipient.

When have you given to others in the past?

My Giving Goals:

1

2

3

Ways to give:

 Give Time

 Volunteer

 Donate or Fundraise

 Spread Kindness

Charities close to my heart:

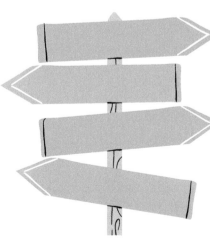

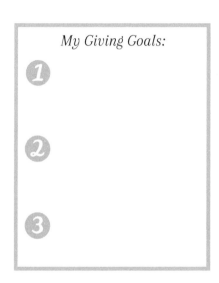

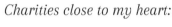

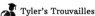 Tyler's Trouvailles

Gratitude

Gratitude is the feeling of being thankful and appreciating what we have. It encourages us to relish positive emotions and experiences, making us feel happy and content.

My Gratitude Jar

Three good things about today:

Draw or write the people, places and things you are grateful for.

Thank You!

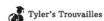

Health

Health encompasses the wellbeing of our physical, mental and social state. Being healthy is about making responsible and informed decisions to benefit our health.

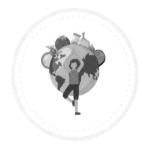
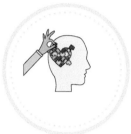

Physical

Our physical body and the way it operates.

Mental

Our wellbeing: emotional, psychological and social.

Social

Our interactions and relationships with others.

Draw or write ways to improve your health and wellness.

Physical, mental and social health all have equal value in achieving positive wellbeing: many things we do can impact more than one element of our health.

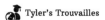

Create your own schedule that prioritises your health.
Try to add an activity each day that supports your
physical, mental and social wellbeing.

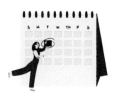

Example:

| WEDNESDAY | 7-7:30 | *Yoga* | ✓ | ✓ | |

My Health Schedule

MONDAY					
TUESDAY					
WEDNESDAY					
THURSDAY					
FRIDAY					
SATURDAY					
SUNDAY					

Reflect...

Did you enjoy your health schedule? Why?
Which activities were successful?
Would you do anything to change your schedule next time?

 Tyler's Trouvailles

Hard-Working

Hard-working describes constant, committed and enthusiastic work.
It requires great effort, shows we are determined and is vital for progres

Why is hard work important?

What does hard work look like?

What do you work hard at?

What do you want to achieve from all your hard work?

What would you like to work harder at?

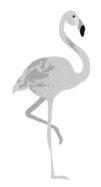

When you work hard, how do you feel?

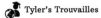

Honesty

Being honest is being completely truthful in what we say and what we do. Honesty is key to building trust and developing positive relationships.

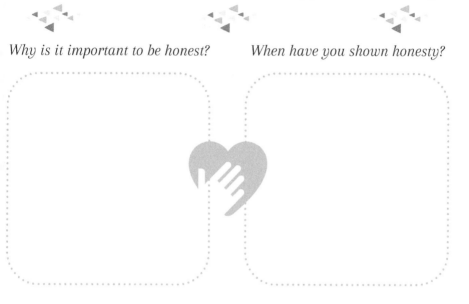

Why is it important to be honest? *When have you shown honesty?*

Write or draw ways to show honesty.

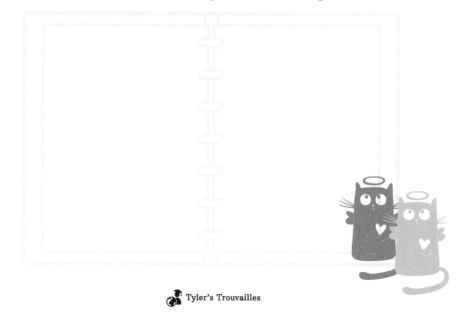

Hope

Hope defines the strong desire for something to happen in the future. It enables us to think positively and optimistically, motivating us to pursue the future we envision and for things to change for the better.

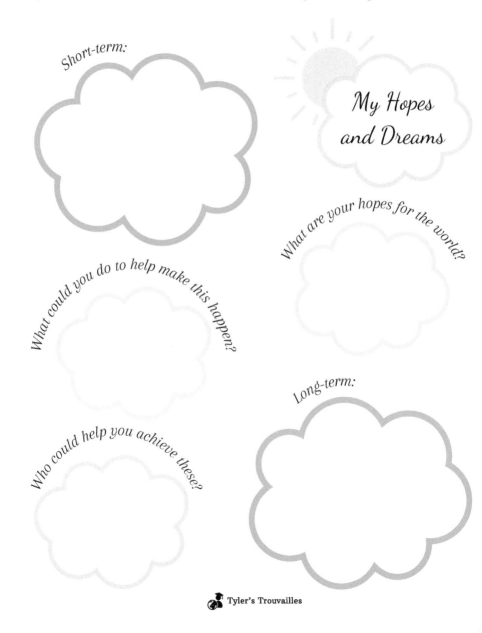

Short-term:

My Hopes and Dreams

What are your hopes for the world?

What could you do to help make this happen?

Long-term:

Who could help you achieve these?

Humility

Humility means being humble and modest. It is important for growth, relationship development and acceptance.

> *I am humble because...*

Colour each square in when you have shown humility in that way.
Write three of your own ways to show humbleness and modesty.

When you lose at something, be happy for the winner.	Let others go before you in a line or queue.	Do something nice for someone, without saying it was you.
Apologise for your mistakes.	Let someone else choose, even if you do not like it or want it for yourself.	Accept criticism from others and learn from it.

Humour

Possessing a sense of humour is vital to living a happy and healthy life. Making someone laugh not only boosts their mood, it can make us more interesting and help us build social bonds with others.

Draw or write some things that make you laugh.

My favourite joke is:

LAUGH S'MORE!

WORRY LESS

I like it because...

SPREAD
HAPPEANESS

HA HA

Fill this box with ways you could make your family or friends laugh.

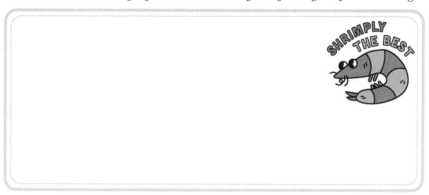

*Create your own jokes on
the post-it notes.*

Remember, making
someone laugh
should not be at the
expense of others.
Always be kind.

SNAILED IT

Independence

Being independent is the freedom and ability to be self-reliant and fulfil things by ourselves. It promotes our confidence and self-esteem.

What could you not do independently when you were younger that you can do now?

Things I can do independently:

What are you looking forward to doing independently in the future?

What might you not be able to do independently when you are older, that you can do now?

Independence is important because...

Individuality

Individuality defines our uniqueness- the different characteristics that form our personality and identity. It embraces freedom and acceptance, allowing us to discover ourselves and personal happiness.

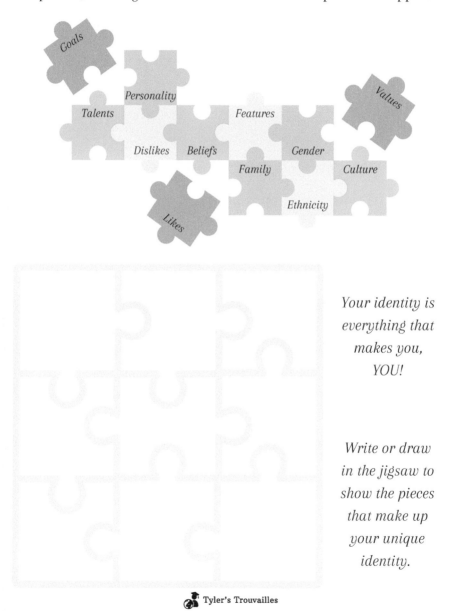

Your identity is everything that makes you, YOU!

Write or draw in the jigsaw to show the pieces that make up your unique identity.

Innovation

Being innovative is all about creating new, original ideas.
Innovation encourages growth and discovery of new opportunities.

If you could create anything, what would your invention be?

My Invention:

Name:

Type:

Purpose:

Target Audience:

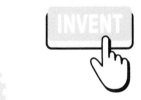

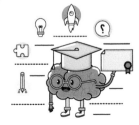

Inspire

Inspiration is the feeling of enthusiasm and motivation we get from someone or something to pursue new or creative ideas. Inspirational people aim to make a difference in the world, showing belief in themselves and others. Inspiration connects us to a positive mindset that can empower us to inspire others too!

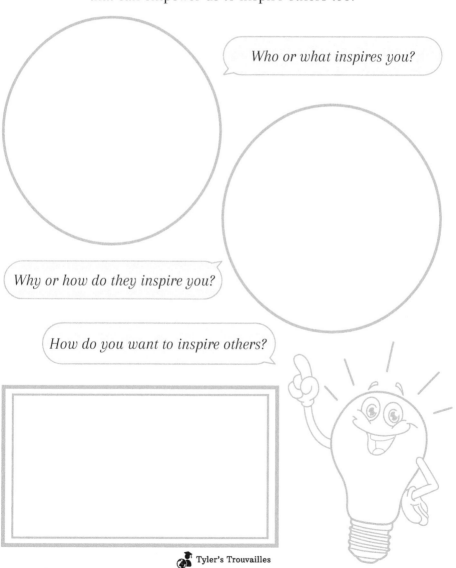

Who or what inspires you?

Why or how do they inspire you?

How do you want to inspire others?

Tyler's Trouvailles

Integrity

Integrity is all about doing the right thing even when it is difficult or when no one is looking. It shows that we are consistent with the values, beliefs and morals we say we hold. Integrity is vital for proving our honesty and building strong, trusting relationships.

How could you show integrity?

Draw a book or film that shows integrity.

Why is it important to always tell the truth?

When have you shown integrity?

Draw facial expressions to reflect the journey of feelings for someone showing integrity in a difficult situation.

Tyler's Trouvailles

Judgement

Judgement describes our evaluation of a situation or thing through combining our personal qualities, experience and knowledge to inform our opinions and decision-making. It is important to spend time considering different perspectives and their consequences within our judgement before making any decisions.

Identify
Identify a time that requires your judgement- this is often followed by the need for a decision to be made.

Think
Consider all viewpoints and assess facts, feelings, experiences and assumptions to make a balanced, fair judgement.

Choose
Evaluate different options, their consequences and prioritise your values- weigh the pros and cons.

Decide
Good judgement needs critical thinking before decision-making: what you are going to say, do and how you are going to act based on everything above?

Reflect
Spend time reflecting on your decisions. Think about how it made you and others feel. What did you learn? Would you change it in any way?

Kindness

Being kind means being considerate, generous and friendly towards ourselves and others. It is essential in boosting morale and positivity.

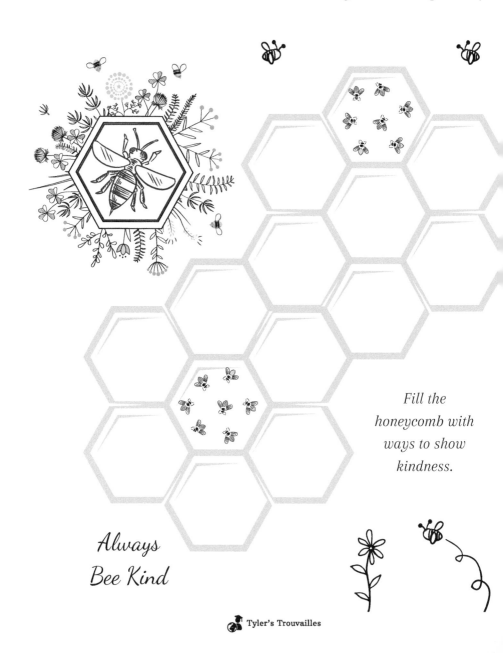

Fill the honeycomb with ways to show kindness.

Always Bee Kind

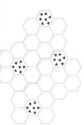
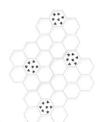

It is as important that we treat ourselves with kindness, as well as others.

We are often quick to speak about ourselves unkindly. Make an effort to switch unkind thoughts into more positive, kinder ones.

Write an unkind phrase you may use towards yourself and sprinkle it with kindness.

Unkind Thoughts...

" I'm stupid. "

Kinder Thoughts...

" I'm learning and trying my best. "

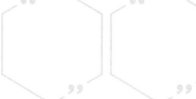

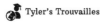

Knowledge

Our knowledge is our personal bank of information and skills that deepens our understanding of the world.

Ways to develop your knowledge:

Learn   *Communicate*   *Research*   *Practice*   *Set Goals*

Use these boxes to organise the knowledge you have gained this year.

English

Maths

Science

Geography

History

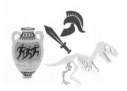

Computing

Languages

Art, Design & Technology

Music & Performing Arts

Physical Education

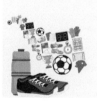

PSHCE & Ethics

Leadership

Leadership is the ability to influence and guide others to do good things and be productive in achieving a goal. It also allows us to have control of our lives, be creative and make things happen through effective teamwork.

Traits of a Good Leader:

What skills should a leader have.

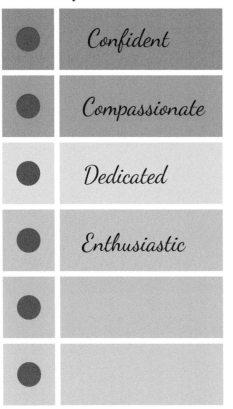

- Confident
- Compassionate
- Dedicated
- Enthusiastic

How are you a good leader?

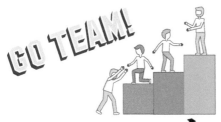

Tyler's Trouvailles

Learning

Learning is the process of gaining knowledge and skills, it enables us to understand the world around us. We learn in many ways, including through study, experiences and communication. Learning boosts our confidence and capabilities, therefore unveils new opportunities.

Your brain produces enough electricity to power a lightbulb!

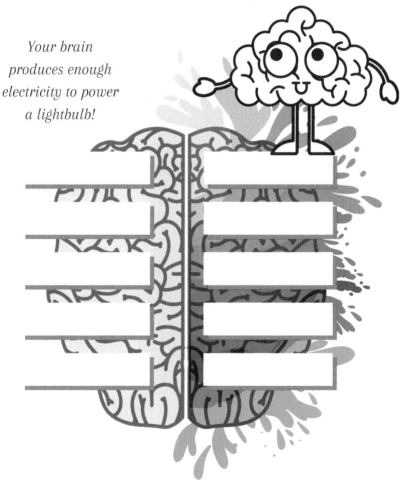

The structure of your brain changes every time you learn or think. Write five things you want to learn this year (left) and five ways you will achieve these learning goals (right).

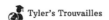

Tyler's Trouvailles

Love

When we really care about something or someone, this is love. It is important to love ourselves, those around us and the world we live in. Love is powerful, it has no limits.

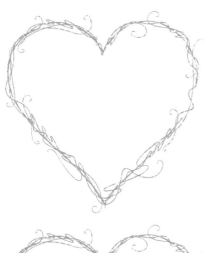

Write or draw some things you love about yourself, someone else or the world and why you love them.

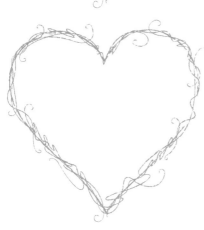

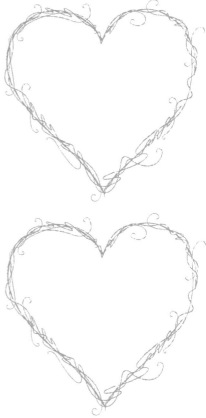

FOLLOW YOUR ♥ Heart

Loyalty

Loyalty defines the commitment we have to others and keeping the promises we make. It strengthens and protects the connections that we have with others.

Why is loyalty important?

What does loyalty look like?

How does it feel to have loyal friends?

Who is loyal to you?

Who are you loyal to?

Open-Mindedness

Being open-minded means being open to new ideas, trying new things and considering different ways of doing things.

It encourages us to look at things from the perspective of others- this can broaden our minds and challenge our thinking.

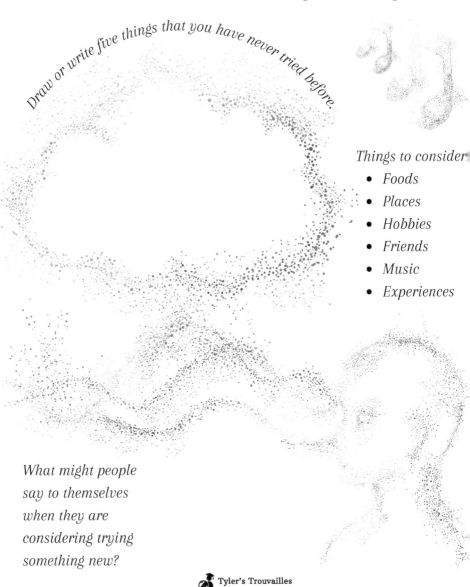

Draw or write five things that you have never tried before.

Things to consider

- *Foods*
- *Places*
- *Hobbies*
- *Friends*
- *Music*
- *Experiences*

What might people say to themselves when they are considering trying something new?

Tyler's Trouvailles

Optimism

Optimism is an attitude that reflects a belief in or hope for the best possible outcome of any situation. Being optimistic helps us become happier, healthier and more successful, as we aim to show our ability to make good things happen.

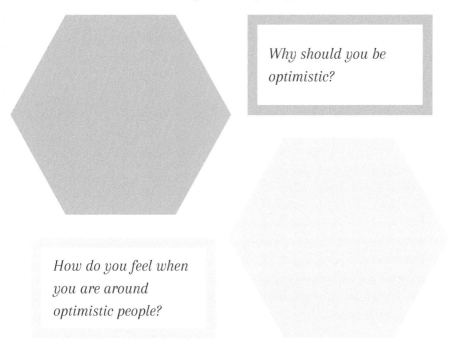

Why should you be optimistic?

How do you feel when you are around optimistic people?

Fill with ways to show optimism:

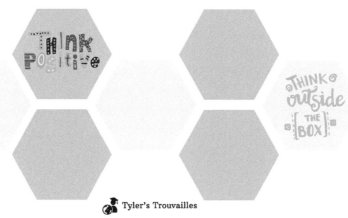

Organisation

Being organised means being efficient and systematic, often in the planning or coordinating of something. Organisation helps us feel in control, allowing us to focus and help prioritise tasks.

Writing lists or schedules is a great way to get organised and plan ahead.

TO DO

Now write them again in order of importance.

People who could help:

DON'T LOSE FOCUS

From __ / __ / __

To   __ / __ / __

Timescale: _____ days/weeks

Tyler's Trouvailles

Stay organised and focused on the steps needed to achieve your goals.

Goal:

Step:	Detail:	Timescale:
1		
2		
3		

Identify your best time of day. Complete the tasks that require more focus and energy during that time.

 Are you an early bird or a night owl?

Try not to do too much at once. Try to complete one thing before moving on to the next. This will give you a sense of achievement and motivate you.

Brain Break Ideas:

Take brain breaks. Try to do this every 20 minutes for just a few minutes. You could take a short walk, make a drink, listen to music, meditate...

Passion

Passion defines a strong feeling of excitement or enthusiasm for something or about doing something that makes us feel good. Passion gives us focus and motivates us to keep learning.

What are you passionate about?

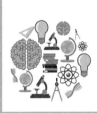

What things do you do related to this passion?

If you could do anything for the rest of your life, what would it be?

What did you love to do when you were younger?

How do you feel when you do something you love?

Patience

Patience defines the ability to wait, accept and tolerate difficult or tedious situations without becoming annoyed or anxious. It plays a vital role in developing our self-control, empathy and resourcefulness.

Why is patience important?   *When might it be difficult*
                                        to have patience?

*List three things you could
do to become more patient:*

Choose a situation that would require patience.

Write or draw an impatient reaction versus patient reaction to this.

Impatient   *Patient*

Vs

Perseverance

Perseverance is the continued effort to achieve goals, even when obstacles arise or when we fail on our journey to success.

How have you shown perseverance in your lifetime?

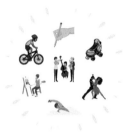

Why is it important to have perseverance?

Failure makes you **resilient** and **strong**.

Failure helps you **learn** and **problem-solve**.

Every failure guides your path to **success**.

Write a positive note to yourself.

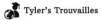 Tyler's Trouvailles

Perspective

Perspective defines our ability to understand a situation from varying points of view. We all have different views on different things, but it is important we respect the views of others. Perspective can reflect the experiences and values of someone, giving us opportunities to learn and understand our differences.

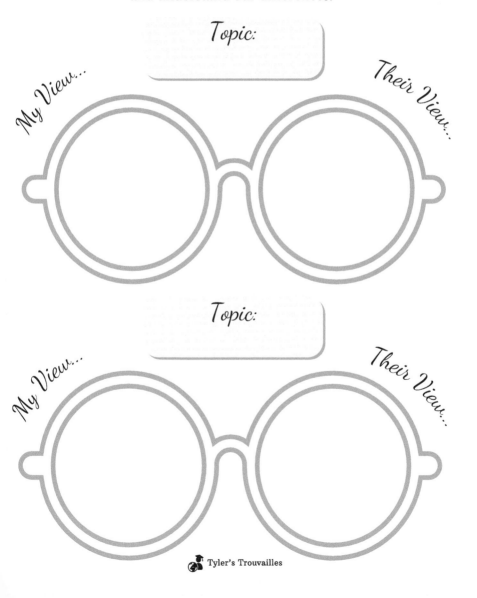

Topic:

My View...

Their View...

Topic:

My View...

Their View...

Positivity

Positivity is the practice of having an optimistic attitude. Positive thinking is a powerful tool for building resilience, developing gratitude and motivating success in all our endeavours.

The best day of your life:

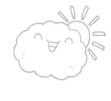

List three good things that have happened today:

Who do you know who is really positive?

Positive thought for today:

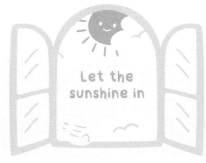

Let the sunshine in

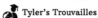

It can sometimes be difficult to find the positives in life, especially when you are having a bad day.

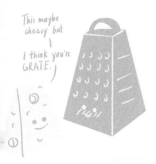

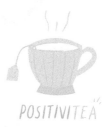

Fill the clouds with some small, positive things that make you feel good.

It could be a song, a person, a smell, a food, a special object...

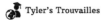 Tyler's Trouvailles

Prudence

Prudence is the ability to make the right choices and judgements. It requires sensibleness and caution in our decision-making, ensuring we consider the consequences of all of our actions.

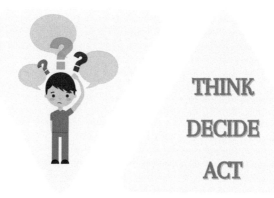

THINK

DECIDE

ACT

Prudence is important because...

Reflect on a time when you wish you had made a better choice or decision

My action looked like this:	*A prudent decision would have been:*

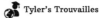

Purpose

Purpose defines the reason why something is done or is the way it is. It can also be a plan that guides life decisions, influences behaviour, shapes goals and creates meaning- it defines who we are and the values we hold. Purpose inspires resilience, compassion and hope.

Three things that give your life meaning:

What are your strengths, values and personal qualities?

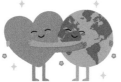

How could these be used to make the world a better place?

Readiness

Readiness means we are willing and prepared for something. When we show readiness, we show we are ready to engage and benefit from knowledge, skills and development.

Readiness to learn checklist:

- ☑ *I follow instructions*
- ☐ *I have the resources I need*
- ☐ *I talk about my ideas and needs*
- ☐ *I share and take turns*
- ☐
- ☐
- ☐

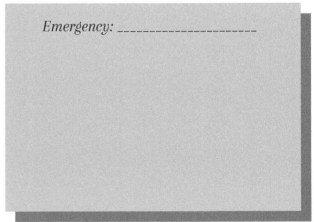

What else shows readiness to learn?

Readiness also includes being prepared when an emergency occurs.

Choose a type of emergency then draw or write six things you would take with you.

Emergency: _____

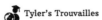

Reliability

Being reliable defines our ability to be trustworthy and responsible in doing something that we have agreed to do- without forgetting or being reminded. It shows that we are consistent and dependable, especially in fulfilling commitments, goals and responsibilities.

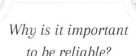

How can you prove you are reliable?

Why is it important to be reliable?

When have you shown reliability?

Why would you want your friends to be reliable?

Respect

Respect is about consideration and admiration of something or someone. Respect is important in developing positive connections and showing acceptance, even when we may not share the same views.

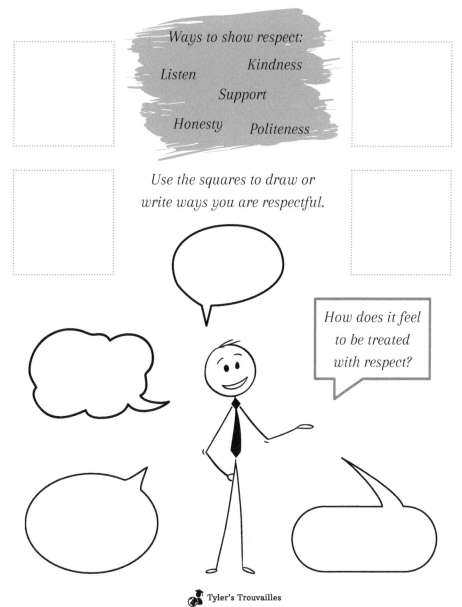

Ways to show respect:

Listen   Kindness

Support

Honesty   Politeness

Use the squares to draw or write ways you are respectful.

How does it feel to be treated with respect?

Tyler's Trouvailles

Responsibility

Being responsible involves knowing expectations and making good choices to fulfil our duties. It involves being accountable for our actions and dependable in making the world a better place.

I am responsible because...

School Responsibilities

What does being responsible at school look like?

World Responsibilities

What are your responsibilities in the wider world?

Home Responsibilities

My favourite chore is...   *My least favourite chore is...*

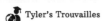

Resilience

Resilience is the ability to cope and 'bounce back' from failure, stress and challenges. Building resilience helps us to overcome obstacles more easily and reduces the chances of us becoming overwhelmed when things change or become difficult.

Ways to develop resilience:

What were their challenges?

How did they overcome them?

Draw someone famous who has shown resilience.

How will their resilience help them in the future?

I showed resilience and 'bounced back' when...

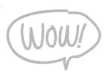

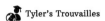

Risk

A positive risk defines a situation that holds the potential of a positive outcome. Even though we may carry feelings of uncertainty or fear, positive risk-taking gives us the opportunity to learn and explore new things, developing our confidence and our ability to cope with challenging situations.

When have you taken a positive risk?

What are the benefits of positive risk-taking?

Remember- some risks can be dangerous and must always be avoided.

 Make a list of positive risks versus negative risks.

Self-Regulation

Self-regulation is the ability to understand and manage our behaviour, emotions, thoughts and reactions. It is crucial in developing our self-awareness, allowing us to become more independent and guide the accomplishment of tasks.

When you are feeling upset, stressed or overwhelmed, focus on your breathing.

Take slow, deep breaths.

BREATHE IN

Pretend you are smelling a flower...

1, 2, 3, 4, 5...

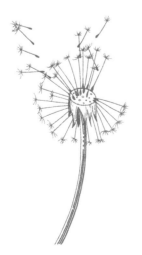

BREATHE OUT

Pretend you are blowing a dandelion...

1, 2, 3, 4, 5...

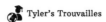

Start at the snake's head.
Slowly, trace your finger or eyes around the snake,
breathing in and out when prompted.

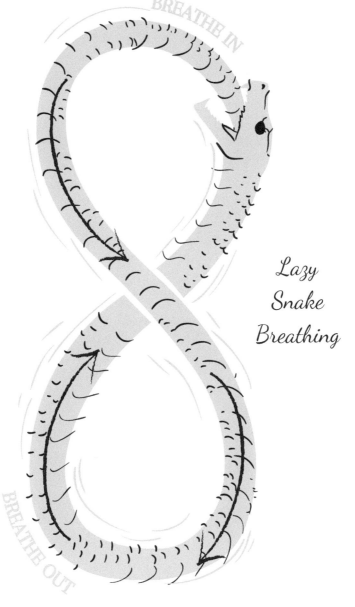

Lazy
Snake
Breathing

Spirituality

Spirituality represents self-discovery: the process of finding and understanding our true selves. This encompasses the realisation of our abilities, beliefs, feelings, character and purpose. Spirituality allows us to make deeper connections with ourselves.

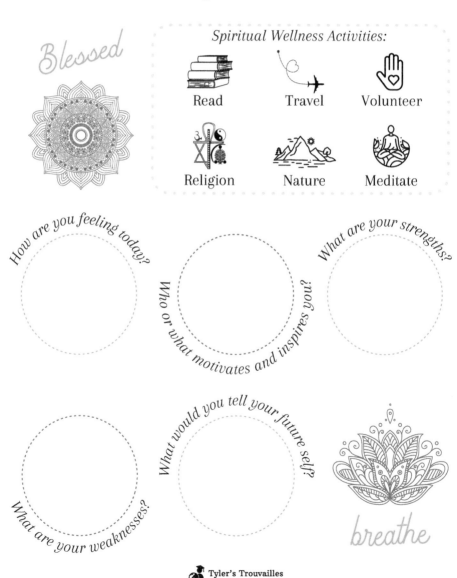

Blessed

Spiritual Wellness Activities:

Read   Travel   Volunteer

Religion   Nature   Meditate

How are you feeling today?

Who or what motivates and inspires you?

What are your strengths?

What are your weaknesses?

What would you tell your future self?

breathe

Teamwork

Teamwork is when we work positively and effectively with other people to support each other in achieving a common goal.
Teamwork utilises different skillsets whilst fostering an enthusiastic and creative working atmosphere.

Draw or write activities that require teamwork:

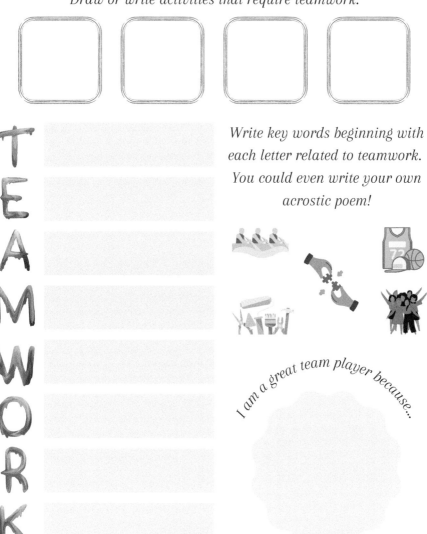

T

E

A

M

W

O

R

K

Write key words beginning with each letter related to teamwork. You could even write your own acrostic poem!

I am a great team player because...

Unity

Unity is all about togetherness. Working together encourages acceptance, respect and allows us to be stronger, as one. Unity is present all around us: at home, in the community, among nature, nationally and all around the world.

Draw or write some examples of unity within the following:

Unity at Home or School:

Unity in the Community:

Unity in Nature:

Wonder

'Wonder' has many meanings. A wonder can mean a person or thing is remarkable. To wonder means we have the desire and curiosity to know something, ultimately encouraging a lifetime of learning.

Choose a topic or go on an adventure...

I notice...

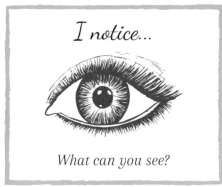

What can you see?

I wonder...

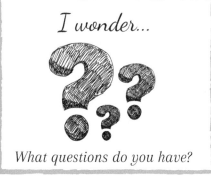

What questions do you have?

I know...

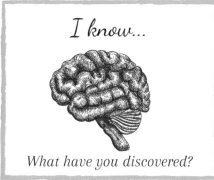

What have you discovered?

Tyler's Trouvailles

Zest

Zest is all about our enthusiasm for life: our energy and vitality. Zest fills us with life-satisfaction and helps spread positivity through performing tasks enthusiastically and wholeheartedly.

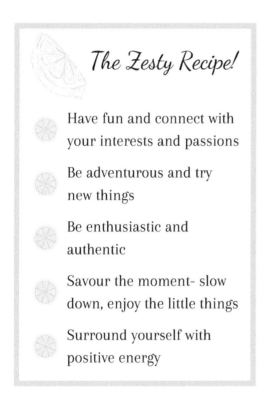

The Zesty Recipe!

- Have fun and connect with your interests and passions
- Be adventurous and try new things
- Be enthusiastic and authentic
- Savour the moment- slow down, enjoy the little things
- Surround yourself with positive energy

What sparks your zest for life?

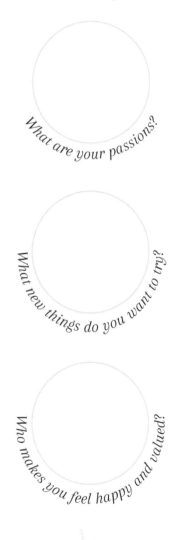

What are your passions?

What new things do you want to try?

Who makes you feel happy and valued?

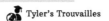

Self-Assessment

Self-assessment enables us to evaluate our strengths and areas for improvement. It is vital for self-awareness, progress and success.

Which skills, values and qualities are your strengths?

How do you know these are your strengths?

Which skills, values and qualities do you need to work on?

Why do you need to work on these?

Which skills, values and qualities do others see in you?
Ask your friends, family, teachers, etc.

What key things have you discovered about life skills, values and qualities

Write three skills, values or qualities you demonstrated last year:	*Write three skills, values or qualities you are prioritising this year:*	*Choose three skills, values or qualities you will focus on next year:*

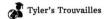 Tyler's Trouvailles

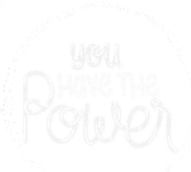

Here are the 66 life skills, values and personal qualities you have studied and reflected on in detail.
Use this page to reflect on their importance to you.
You could highlight, circle, tick those significant to you or even number them in order of importance!

Acceptance	Freedom	Open-Mindedness
Accountability	Friendship	Optimism
Adaptability	Giving	Organisation
Ambition	Gratitude	Passion
Appreciation	Health	Patience
Awareness	Hard-Working	Perseverance
Balance	Honesty	Perspective
Calm	Hope	Positivity
Compassion	Humility	Prudence
Courage	Humour	Purpose
Creativity	Independence	Readiness
Communication	Individuality	Reliability
Confidence	Innovation	Respect
Connection	Inspire	Responsibility
Curiosity	Integrity	Resilience
Determination	Judgement	Risk
Discipline	Kindness	Self-Regulation
Diversity	Knowledge	Spirituality
Empathy	Leadership	Teamwork
Equality	Learning	Unity
Fairness	Love	Wonder
Forgiveness	Loyalty	Zest

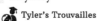 Tyler's Trouvailles

Unwind

Take a Mindful Moment

Take the time to be aware of your senses in different places and at different moments.

Draw or write in the boxes to identify what you can see, hear, smell, taste and touch.

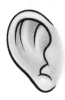

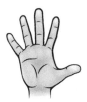

Self-Care

Self-care is all about prioritising and maintaining a healthy relationship with ourself. It is vital for improving our focus, strengthening relationships and motivating us to live our best life.

Fill the squares with ways you can look after yourself.

Listen to music

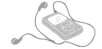

Read a book

Get creative

Take a walk

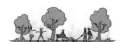

Have a bath

Take a nap

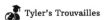

My Self-Care Priorities This Year...

Make notes in each section of your self-care priorities- this could include activities, events or things you would like to achieve to support each area of your self-care this year.

Physical   Mental

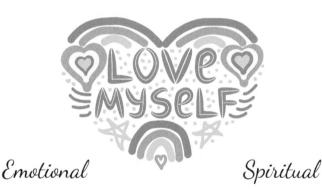

Emotional   Spiritual

Yoga

Yoga is a calming form of exercise that focuses on developing strength, flexibility and mindful breathing. Here are some simple yoga poses- try holding each of these for ten to thirty seconds.

Be aware of your surroundings, ensure you are wearing appropriate exercise clothing and drink lots of water.
Never force yourself into a pose.

Be mindful of your breath- breathe in for a count of five, breathe out for a count of five. Feel your tummy rising and falling...

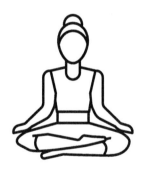

EASY POSE

Sit on the floor and cross your legs. Rest your hands on your knees. Keep your back straight, relax your shoulders. Take slow, deep breaths.

BUTTERFLY POSE

Stay in a seated position. Bring the soles of your feet together in front of you. Sit up straight and tall. Hold your ankles, then allow your knees to fall out to either side. Gently, lean forwards to fold into the pose.

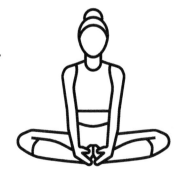

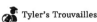 Tyler's Trouvailles

CHILD'S POSE

Sit back on your heels. Slowly, bring your forehead down in front of your knees. Rest your arms alongside your body, palms facing upwards.

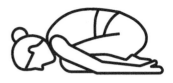

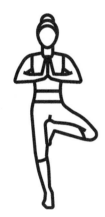

TREE POSE

Stand on one leg. Bend the other knee and place the sole of your foot on your inner calf or thigh. Keep your posture strong and tall. Put your palms together- try reaching them above your head. Hold for ten seconds, then swap legs.

UPWARD SALUTE POSE

Stand with your feet parallel and slightly apart. Focus on your posture- back straight, shoulders relaxed and balanced. Reach your arms up, keeping your shoulders away from your ears.

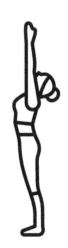

Namaste

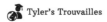

Drawing Development

Create a simple design in the first box and then develop it, step by step.
You could always try this in reverse, starting with your finished design
and breaking it down into its simplest form.

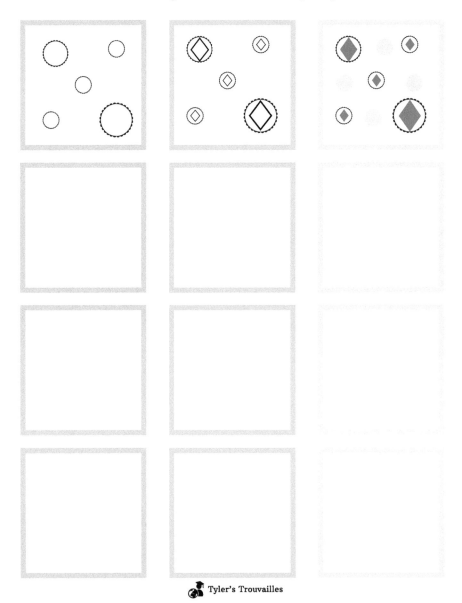

Circle Search

Draw as many circular or spherical objects you can find or know.

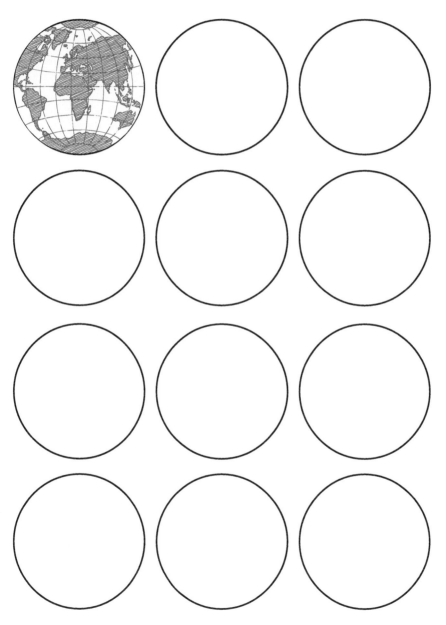

Mirror Mirror

Can you draw the other half of each design?

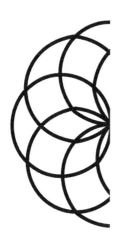

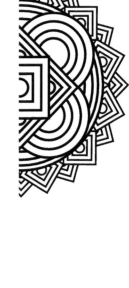

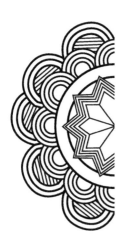

Doodle Breathing

Trace the lines with your pencil- let your breathing guide you. Match the speed of your breathing to the speed of your drawing. Inhale as you go up and exhale as you go down.

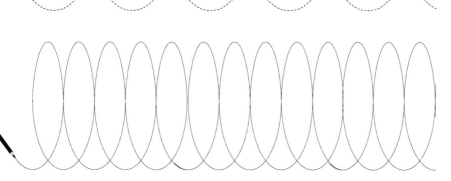

Experiment creating your own. Aim to inhale and exhale for longer. This will make you more relaxed and in control of your breathing.

Imagination Creations

Let your imagination run wild!
Use the shapes and outlines to create your own mini masterpieces!

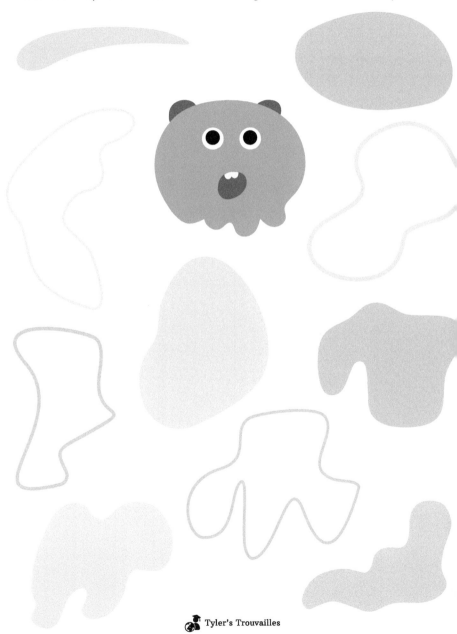

Animal Antics

What is your favourite animal?
Draw it in its natural habitat.

What facts do you know
about this animal?

If I were an animal, I would be...

because...

What would you look like?

Under the Sea

Design your own aquarium.

How many different species of fish and plants could you include?

Woodland Wandering

Can you design a new habitat for these lost woodland animals?

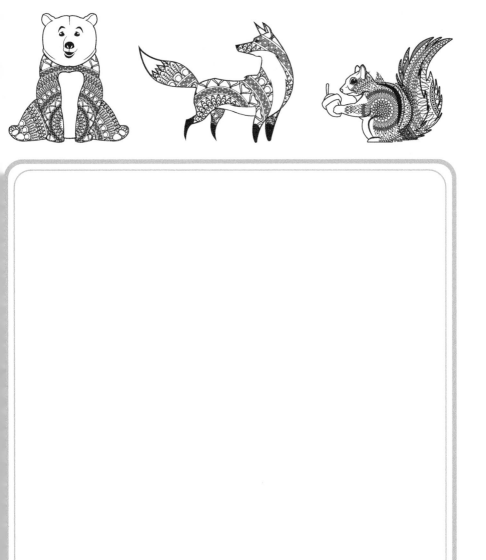

Tech Check

Technology can be great for helping us connect, learn and wind down, however, it can also consume so much of our time without us even realising. It is really important that we take time away from screens and technology- enjoy being in the moment.

When do you use technology the most?

Try turning your phone off for a few hours or for a whole day!

What technology is around you?

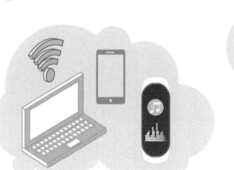

Spend an evening without technology- colour, read, spend time with family, cook...

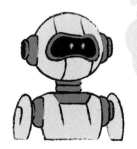

Be aware of when you use technology and how long for- limit this and make it purposeful.

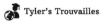 Tyler's Trouvailles

Fill the clouds with **technology-free** *ways you could spend your time.*

*What is your favourite thing to do (that **does not** require technology) and why?*

Treehouse Timeout

Meditation scripts are a great way to be mindful and relax. They are short exercises that encourage us to use our imagination and take our mind to a calm and peaceful place.

Use this space to draw your dream treehouse.

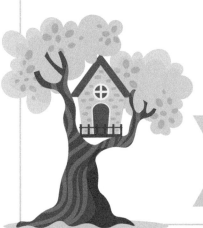

You can read this script aloud in a quiet, gentle voice or politely ask someone to do this for you.

1. *Get your body into a comfortable position and close your eyes.*

2. *Slowly take three deep breaths, in through your nose and out through your mouth. Feel your tummy rising and falling.*

3. *Take notice of your legs and feet. Relax them. Let them become heavy. Imagine the air surrounding you relaxes everything it touches.*

4. *Gently breathe in... and out. Feel the air entering and leaving your body. Now release the tension you are holding. Relax your neck, tummy, chest and shoulders.*

5. *Pay attention to your arms and fingers. Feel how relaxed you are.*

6. *Now imagine you are standing in front of a tall tree. This tree has deep roots. It is grounded. Branches reach in every direction.*

7. *Wrapped within the branches lies a treehouse. Your very own treehouse. Imagine what your treehouse would look like.*

8. *What makes your treehouse special? What makes it your peaceful, safe space? You can add all your favourite things.*

9. *Allow yourself to travel inside the treehouse. Fill your treehouse with everything that makes you feel good. Relaxed. Let go of all your thoughts and worries.*

10. *When you are ready, take a deep breath and imagine you are standing, looking up at your treehouse again.*

11. *Be still. Now gently rub your hands together for a count of five. 1, 2, 3, 4, 5. Carefully, place them over your eyes.*

12. *Take three deep breaths. In... and out. Slowly, open your eyes and bring your attention back to the present moment.*

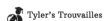

Scribble Story

Sometimes it can be difficult to say exactly how we feel, but drawing can be easier for us to reflect on our feelings.

Complete your scribble story at different points in the day.

You can scribble, write feelings, emotions or even write the name of someone who made you feel a certain way.

Example: Cold   Content   Frustrated
Excited   Sam   Creative

MON

TUES

WED

THUR

FRI

SAT

SUN

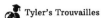

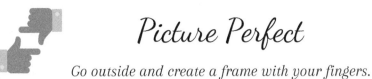

Picture Perfect

Go outside and create a frame with your fingers.
This could be a wide-lens (capturing a view) or a close-up lens (focusing on a specific thing, like a plant). Draw what you have captured.

Passing Thoughts

Thoughts are very powerful, constant and can have a huge impact on how we feel. It is important to take time to pay attention to these thoughts and consider their impact on us.

Sit in a calm and quiet space. What are your thoughts in this exact moment?

Some thoughts pass through our minds very quickly, some bring back memories, others can cause us to worry.

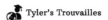

Sleeping Soundly

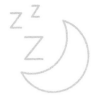

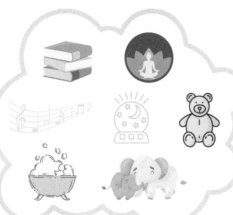

Sleep improves
memory, behaviour,
attention, learning
and health.

*What do you do to
help you sleep?*

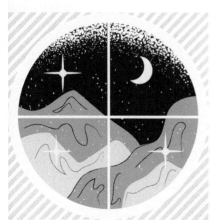

Out of this World

Draw what you think you might discover if you left Earth.

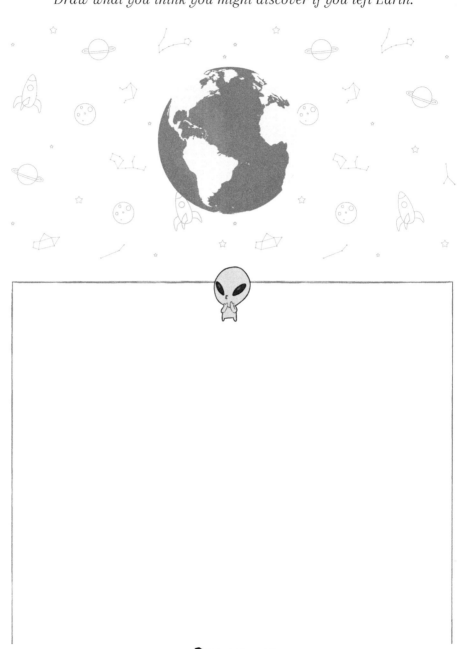

Cloud-Gazing

Lay down and look at the sky. What can you see? Gaze at a cloud, what does it look like? Ask a friend, can they see the same shape or do they perceive it differently? Trace the cloud with your finger, then draw it. Write what you and your friends think it looks like.

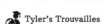

Wondrous Wandering

Spend time wandering your local green spaces. Not only is this good exercise, it is a great mindful activity to help you feel relaxed and be grateful for what life and nature has to offer.

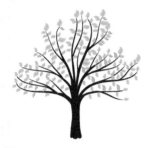

Take deep breaths. Walk slowly. Focus on each and every step.
What is your body doing? How are you holding yourself?
Think about what each body part is doing as you walk.

Look around you. Take time to watch movement around you. Focus on detail. What do you notice? What texture and scent do certain plants have? What is below you? What is above you? What season is it? How do you know?

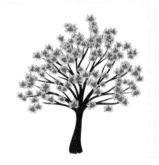

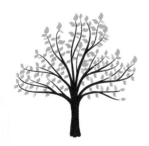

Now reflect on each of your senses. What can you see? What sounds can you hear? What smells fill the air? Can you taste anything? How do you feel? Is there anything you can touch?

Use this space to draw and reflect on your experience.

Shadow Silhouettes

A shadow is formed when light is blocked- the outline or shape is called silhouette. Though shadows often have a similar shape to the object block the light, angles and distance can impact what the shadow looks like.

Choose an object and cast a shadow on the page. Trace around the shadow with a pencil.

What does your shadow drawing look like? Can you turn it into something different?

Food for Thought

Different foods can boost our mood and bring us comfort.
Baking and cooking can be fun, relaxing activities that can refocus
our minds and reward us with something tasty!

Create your dream menu.

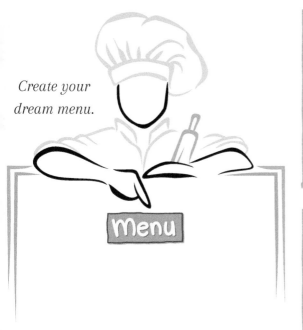

What are your favourite foods?

What do you enjoy baking or cooking?

How do you feel when you are making this?

Tyler's Trouvailles

Sensational Seasons

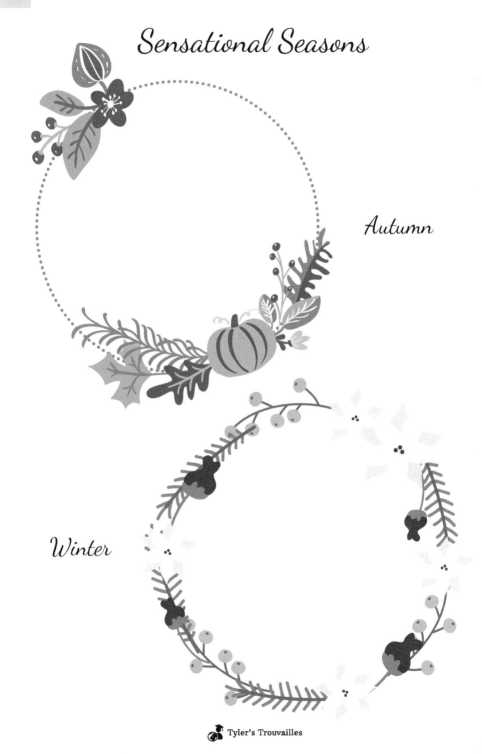

Autumn

Winter

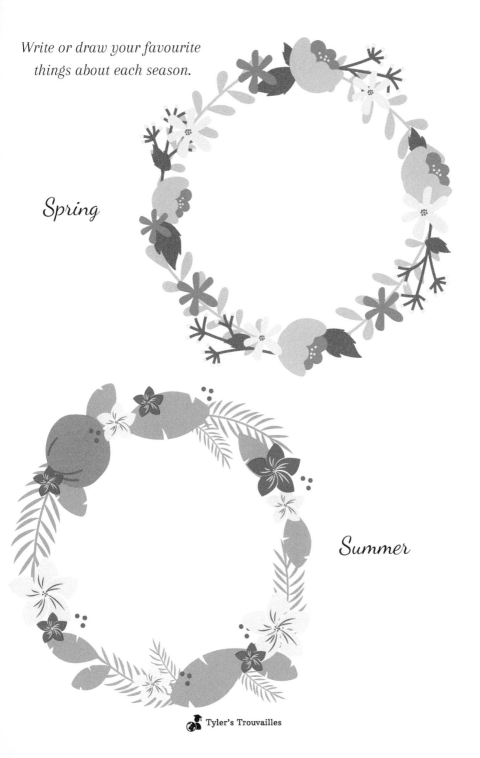

Write or draw your favourite things about each season.

Spring

Summer

Tyler's Trouvailles

Wonderful World

Our planet is awe-inspiring- its diversity offers a wealth of opportunities to develop our learning and love for the world we live in.

On the next seven pages, you will find the seven continents of the world. Fill these pages with words, drawings and facts about each of them. Remember to include your knowledge of countries, cities, famous landmarks, flags, wildlife, culture, traditions, foods, sports, history and geography.

Can you name the seven continents in order of size, starting with the largest?

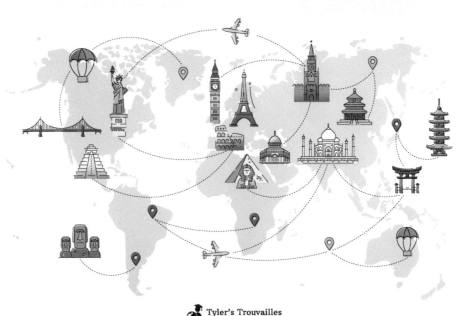

Tyler's Trouvailles

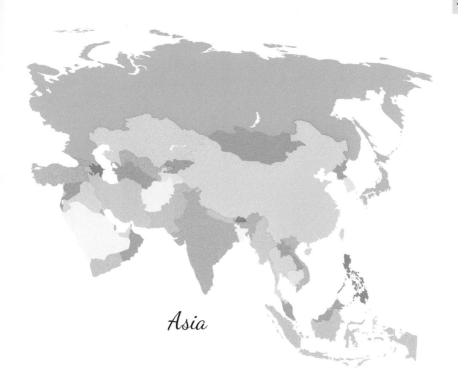

Asia

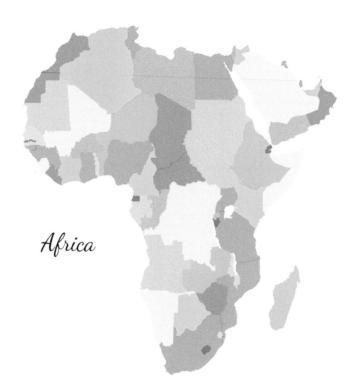

Africa

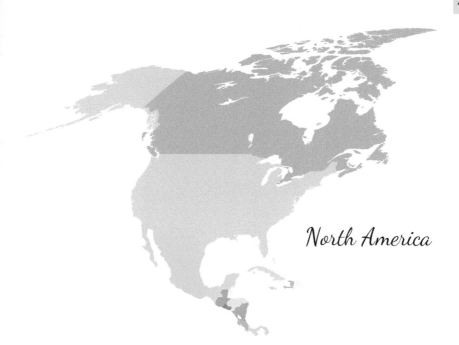

North America

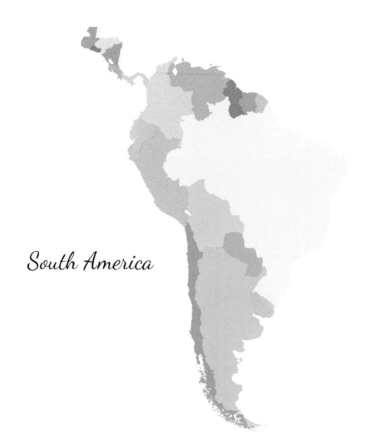

South America

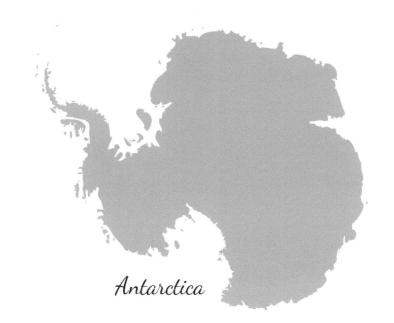

Antarctica

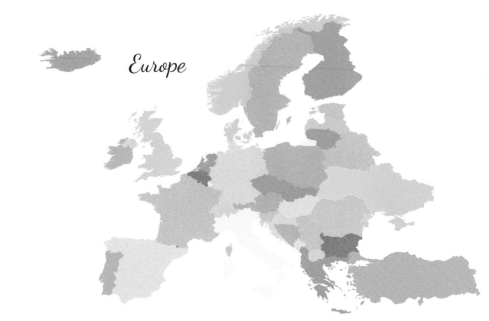

Europe

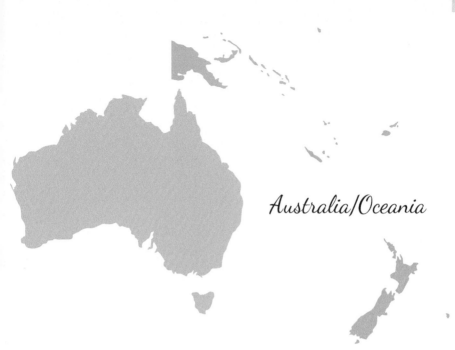

Australia/Oceania

Alphabet Scavenger Hunt

1. *Find an item beginning with each letter of the alphabet- this could be at home, school or wherever your adventure takes you!*
Colour each letter of the alphabet once you have found something.
2. *Fill each page with words and drawings of as many different people, places and things, beginning with that letter, as you can.*

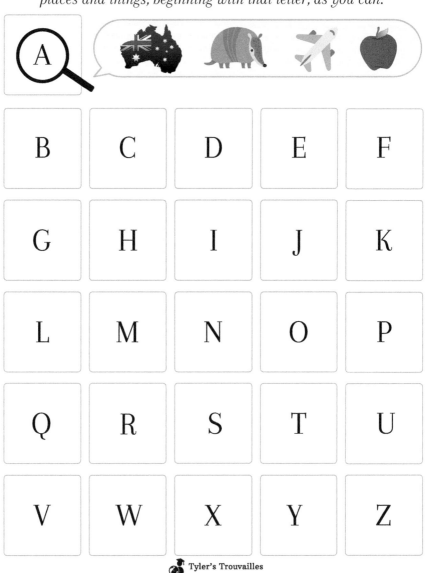

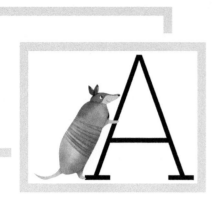

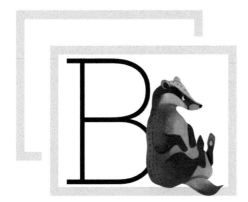

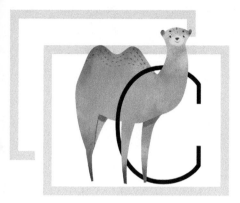

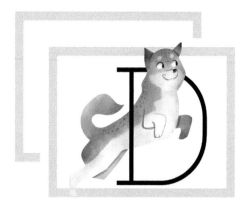

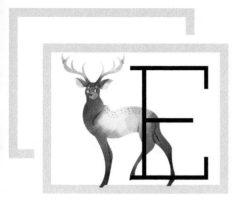

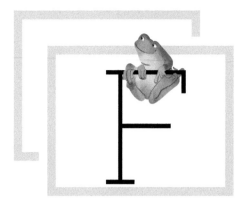

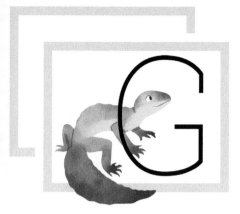

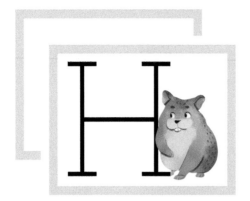

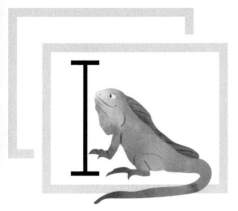

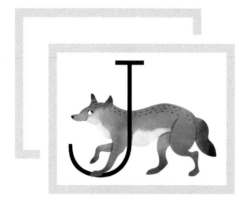

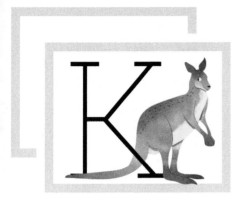

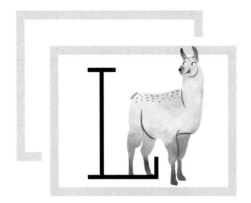

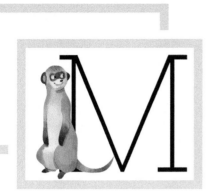

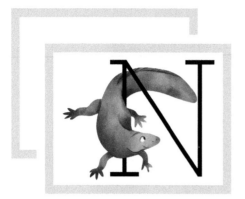

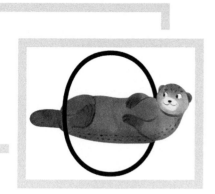

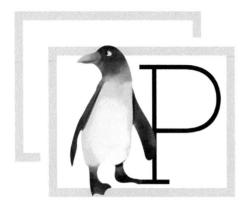

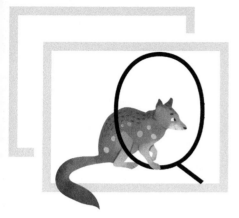

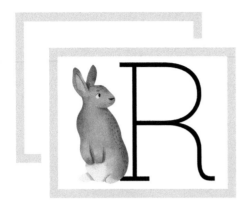

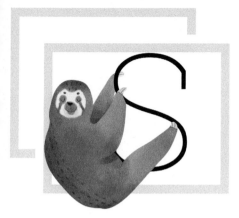

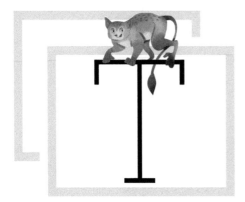

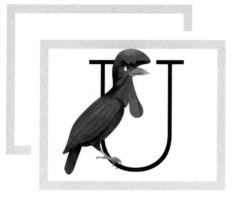

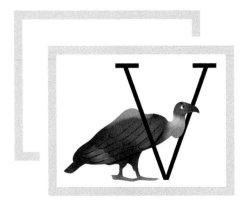

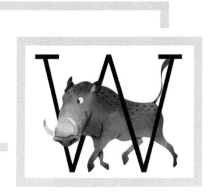

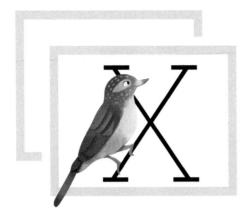

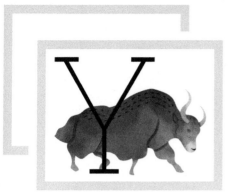

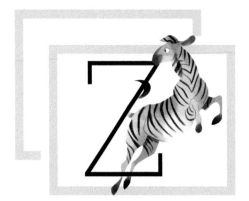

Delightful Doodles

Sometimes we just want to put pen to paper and see where our mind takes us. This is a great way to relax and appreciate the present moment.

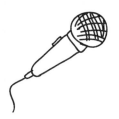

On the next twelve pages, there are dedicated doodle pages- one for each month of the year.

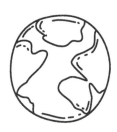

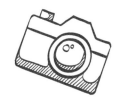

You can add to these throughout the year- you could use them on the month itself or fill with things which remind you of that month... it is completely up to you!

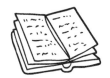

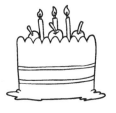

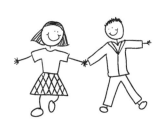

Sit comfortably. Consider your posture.

Take time to focus. Do not rush.

Doodle Tips!

Focus on sensations. How does the pen feel, sound, draw?

Be creative. Try different colours, patterns or something new!

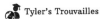

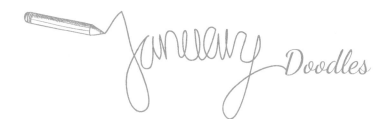

January Doodles

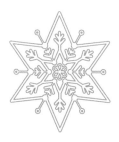

February Doodles

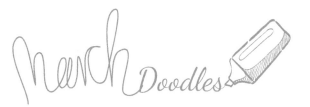

March Doodles

April Doodles

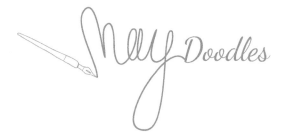

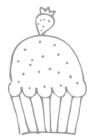

June Doodles

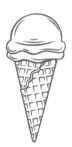

July Doodles

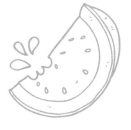

August Doodles

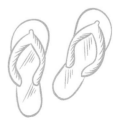

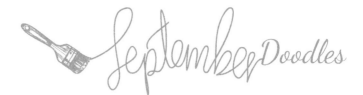

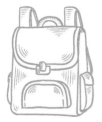

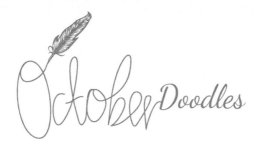

October Doodles

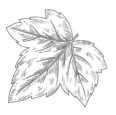

November Doodles

December Doodles

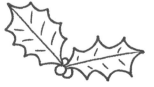

Image Credits

Every reasonable effort has been made to acknowledge all copyright holders, namely the creative contributors via Canva.com. Any errors or omissions that may have occurred are inadvertent. Anyone with any copyright queries are invited to write directly to the publisher to ensure full acknowledgement may be included in subsequent editions of the work. *Tyler's Trouvailles* admires and thanks all artists for sharing their talents and for their dedication to their creative works.

©a-arrow via Canva.com; ©Abi Afandi via Canva.com; ©aidenopoly via Canva.com; ©Aimagenarium via Canva.com; ©akimomia via Canva.com; ©Aleksander via Canva.com; ©alexanderkonoplyov via Canva.com; ©Alisa Foytik via Canva.com; ©Allies Interactive via Canva.com; ©Andres Rodriguez via Canva.com; ©angelainthefields via Canva.com; ©Anugraha Design via Canva.com; ©Aplum Studio via Canva.com; ©ArtnerDluxe via Canva.com; ©Aurielaki via Canva.com; ©barsrsind via Canva.com; ©beaandbloom.com via Canva.com; ©Belle's via Canva.com; ©blankstock via Canva.com; ©BNPDesignStudio via Canva.com; ©bomsymbols via Canva.com; ©Boykopictures via Canva.com; ©Brittva via Canva.com; ©Canva via Canva.com; ©Canva Layouts via Canva.com; ©Canva Original Graphics via Canva.com; ©Chasnutisindustries via Canva.com; ©Chikovnaya via Canva.com; ©christianhorz via Canva.com; ©Clker-Free-Vector-Images via Canva.com; ©Color Vectors via Canva.com; ©creativemahira via Canva.com; ©creativepriyanka via Canva.com; ©Crocus Paperi via Canva.com; ©curvabezier via Canva.com; ©DAPA Images via Canva.com; ©Davids47 via Canva.com; ©dDara via Canva.com; ©Delwar Hossain via Canva.com; ©DesignbyCheyney via Canva.com; ©djvstock via Canva.com; ©djvstock2 via Canva.com; ©DKDesignz via Canva.com; ©dmytrokozyrskyi via Canva.com; ©doloves via Canva.com; ©Dominik Schröder, 2015 via Canva.com; ©Dooder via Canva.com; ©elenadrozhzhina via Canva.com; ©Elionas via Canva.com; ©Ellette Lorelei via Canva.com; ©Ember Studio via Canva.com; ©EncoderXSolutions via Canva.com; ©Eucalyp via Canva.com; ©Febrina Noor's Images via Canva.com; ©feelisgood via Canva.com; ©FlatIcons via Canva.com; ©florintenica via Canva.com; ©Fusion Books via Canva.com; ©galynatymonko via Canva.com; ©GDJ via Canva.com; ©GeoImages via Canva.com; ©grebeshkov via Canva.com; ©greenpic.studio via Canva.com; ©grmarc via Canva.com; ©grmarc2 via Canva.com; ©gstudioimagen via Canva.com; ©gstudioimagen2 via Canva.com; ©Hea Poh Lin via Canva.com; ©Iconika Pro via Canva.com; ©icons via Canva.com; ©Icons8 via Canva.com; ©Iconsolid via Canva.com; ©iconsy via Canva.com;©igorkrasnoselskyi via Canva.com; ©ivandesign via Canva.com; ©jemastock via Canva.com;

Tyler's Trouvailles

Hello, Tyler Here...

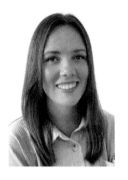

Thank you for your time in engaging with my book and for being part of *Tyler's Trouvailles* journey in *'Inspiring and empowering a generation of self-love and world love'* through *'Discovering the people, places and things that make you feel blessed'.*

My ultimate life goal is to make a difference. Big or small. Making a difference has always been a priority of mine: through my career, volunteering, charitable contributions and lifestyle choices. As a Primary School Teacher and World Explorer, I aim to inspire and share my passion for education, positive wellbeing and the world we live in. Education is the most empowering force in the universe, without it we would have no knowledge, no understanding and no individuality. Let's continue to learn inspire and grow together- stay tuned at tylerstrouvailles.com and on social media @tylerstrouvailles

Vision

Inspiring and empowering a generation of self-love and world love.

Mission

Discovering the people, places and things that make you feel blessed.

Values

Learn

Discovering is learning. Learning is indispensable and lifelong- it is imperative for personal development, contentment and fulfilment.

Connect

Innovating positive relationships to explore and appreciate our world of diversity, shaping a generation of acceptance, unity and understanding.

Inspire

Sparking curiosity and awakening the mind to a world of new possibilities, limitless aspirations and transformative life experiences.

Impact

Believing that passion, accountability and integrity leads to a positive influence and change in ourselves, others and the world.

Tyler's Trouvailles

'No place is the same, nor will it be experienced by anyone in the same way. Open your mind and your heart, the world will change you.' — Tyler